The 17 Day Plan
to Stop Aging

ALSO BY DR. MIKE MORENO

The 17 Day Diet

The 17 Day Diet Journal

The 17 Day Diet Cookbook

The 17 Day Plan to Stop Aging

DR. MIKE MORENO

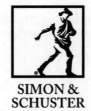

**SIMON &
SCHUSTER**

London · New York · Sydney · Toronto · New Delhi

A CBS COMPANY

First published in Great Britain by Simon & Schuster UK Ltd, 2012
A CBS COMPANY

1 3 5 7 9 10 8 6 4 2

Simon & Schuster UK Ltd
1st Floor
222 Gray's Inn Road
London WC1X 8HB

www.simonandschuster.co.uk

Simon & Schuster Australia, Sydney
Simon & Schuster India, New Delhi

A CIP catalogue record for this book is available
from the British Library

ISBN: 978-1-47111-490-8
ISBN: 978-1-47111-491-5 (ebook)

Printed and bound by CPI Group (UK) Ltd, Croydon, CR0 4YY

This book is dedicated to my loving and supportive family and friends, to my incredible patients who inspire me every day, and to the millions of people around the world who used The 17 Day Diet *as a springboard to reclaim their health and vitality. I am so proud of each and every one of you who empowered yourself to lose weight. It brings me such honor and joy to know that I played a role in your success.*

NOTE TO READERS

ACKNOWLEDGMENTS

I appreciate Maggie Greenwood-Robinson and Lisa Clark for their contribution to this book. I'd also like to thank the many people who were instrumental in bringing this project to life and the entire amazing team at Free Press, for their passion, creativity, and dedication. I sincerely hope that the information within these pages will help millions of people live longer, happier, healthier lives. It's never too late to start paving the way to 100 happy, healthy years!

CONTENTS

INTRODUCTION

My Approach to Living 100 Happy, Healthy Years

Every year, every month, every day, every hour, every minute, down to every single second that you are alive, you are getting older. Your body is probably undergoing age-related changes that all too often lead to less energy, painful joints, droopy skin, unsightly wrinkles, graying or thinning hair, and overall declining health. But what if I told you that getting older and the physical process of aging don't have to be so closely entwined? And what if you had the power to slow down the aging of your body systems . . . so much so that you could actually live to see, and more importantly, *enjoy* your 100th birthday, or beyond? Allow me to explain.

I have a different way of looking at health and longevity: one that is organized according to the way your body is organized, and that is by body systems. By "body systems" I mean the networks of organs and tissues that work together to keep you alive—your circulatory system, nervous system, respiratory system, immune system, reproductive system, and so forth. The systems in your body typically begin to decline at around age 20, a piece of knowledge given to us by the Baltimore Longitudinal Study of Aging. Focus on the well-being of those systems—and the lifestyle changes you can make to postpone their aging—and you're on your way to living 100 healthy years.

As a family practice physician, I like to zero in on all of those different body systems early, before someone even has symptoms, so I can identify the risk factors that may affect a person. Then it's my job to intervene before the person develops a particular disease.

All of our body systems are interrelated in fascinating ways, many of which I'll discuss in this book. So, if you take care of even a few body systems, all the systems benefit, and your reward is rejuvenated health and longevity.

Even in advanced age, some body systems can still remain robust with the right treatment. The disease-free heart, for example, can actually get stronger with age; in a person free of heart disease, especially one who exercises regularly, the cardiac output is just about the same in old age as it is in a younger person.

The lungs, on the other hand, lose their elasticity, making it harder to fill them with as much air as when they were young. Joints stiffen as we get older. Exercise, however, can increase the lungs' capacity and counteract stiffness, both of which make a huge difference in your well-being. In other words, getting off your butt now—no matter what age you are—can make all the difference in how your body ages for years to come.

I'll start you on the longevity road by showing you how to "restore" your primary systems: your heart (circulatory), lungs (respiratory), and brain (nervous). I call them "primary" because they're the ones most responsible for keeping you alive. Your heart beats, your lungs breathe, and your brain, well, it controls just about everything in your body. Plus, they're the most susceptible to factors that cause aging. Thus, the initial work of anti-aging must start with these systems, in what I call *Cycle 1: Restore*. I'll give you simple but health-changing strategies and prescriptions to help you restore those systems, stop health problems before they start, and begin to feel better right away. And by "right away," I mean in 17 days flat.

Next, I'll introduce you to the secondary systems of the body: your immune, digestive, endocrine, and musculoskeletal systems. They're support systems, governed by your primary systems. Much of what keeps you well and vital is found in how healthy these support systems are. They protect you, give you energy, and contribute to your overall well-being. It takes a number of strategies to rebuild, or shore up, these systems, and you'll learn how to do that in *Cycle 2: Rebuild*.

Cycle 3: Refine focuses on fine-tuning your subsystems: the delicate reproductive (male and female) and urinary systems. When these systems are working at their peak, you'll feel sexy, vibrant, and really at the top of your game. I've got several measures to help you "refine" these systems so you can be all that you deserve to be, every single day.

Finally, I offer *Cycle 4: Renew*. It's designed to help you create harmony between your health, your environment, and your lifestyle. The steps you take in this final cycle will also protect the progress you've made in the first three cycles.

Some of you may need to work through all four cycles; others may need to work on fewer. It all depends on your current state of health. And how do you gauge that? For every system of the body, I've developed 14-point assessments to help you. You'll instantly find out where you stand on the road to 100 happy, healthy years. Don't skip the assessments; your scores tell you which aspects of your health you must concentrate on to maximize your longevity.

There are also 17-day plans for each cycle. These plans tell you exactly what to do each day to start transforming your systems. Folks, this is a no-brainer, no-guesswork deal that gets you on your way toward that magic, but achievable, number: 100.

I'll be candid here. I used to think I didn't want to live to be 100. I feared that I might be chained to a wheelchair or hospital bed, with no real quality of life. Then again, when I was 25 years old I wasn't particularly keen on reaching my present age of 43, imagining that 43 was pretty darn old. Now I know better. There is still so much to live for, especially when I know that I can be living for it in a healthy and comfortable way.

I know you have doubts. Like many of my patients, perhaps you think it's too late for you. But I don't think it is *ever* too late. Even if you're already middle-aged with some health issues, you have a much better chance of reaching 90 or even 100 if you follow the guidelines I will set out here. Not only can you be free of heart disease and stroke, but also from a number of other chronic illnesses, including cancer. What if you already have health issues such as diabetes or heart disease? You can still live 100 healthy years if you change certain behaviors and correct poor lifestyle choices. But don't panic. The changes I'm talking about are super simple, and will become second-nature good habits in no time at all.

I want us all to strive for that magical number and adjust our lives to get there. In my 20s, I became aware of the importance of living healthfully. I focused on running with more intensity and tried to maintain a regular schedule of physical activity, even when the demands of med school left me drained. I changed my diet as best I could to focus more on natural foods. And I tried to manage my schedule to include more relaxation, fun, and joy. Each of us is capable of enhancing our own health to the point of living 100 years. Is it worth the effort that these changes require? I believe so.

PART ONE

• •

Stop Your
Aging Clock

You've heard the expression "all roads lead to Rome." Well, this was true in ancient days, after the Romans constructed 50,000 miles of paved road and each road led back to the city. Thousands of years and a zillion research studies later, we know that the roads leading to longevity all lead back to our physical bodies—more specifically, to the way we take care of key body systems. In the first part of this book, you'll learn how to stop your body from revolting against you and instead reverse many of the things that are conspiring to age you.

Those "conspirators" are the five factors of aging—the real nitty-gritty of what's causing you to get older. The fascinating aspect of these factors is that you can control them! That's right. I'll give you strategies to stop Father Time in his tracks and show you how to build an anti-aging base that will send him packing.

I'll be the first to admit that staying young and vital takes some work, and not everyone might be willing to put forth the effort, so I'm making it as easy as I can. If you do just a few of the measures I recommend here—

none takes longer than minutes a day—well, say hello to 100 happy, healthy years!

By dedicating yourself to reaching a higher level of health, you're also becoming a role model to others who have yet to walk the same road. So, keep walking! Improve your life and you'll improve the lives of those around you. I'll be by your side the whole way . . . helping you live 100 healthy years through strategies and suggestions that really work and are super-easy to integrate into your life. Let's go!

CHAPTER 1

Five Factors of Aging

Has it happened to you? Sagging skin. Thinning hair. Brittle bones. Love handles. Forgetfulness. Indescribable aches and pains. It's hard to believe that would happen to robust, youthful you. Until it does. Poof: You're old. Ick.

How does it happen? In the past, anti-aging experts looked at aging as a cumulative process, meaning that over time, our bodies deteriorate. But the latest research indicates that aging could really be an active, not passive, process brought on by five key *controllable* factors. Notice I say "controllable." Yes, aging is largely within our control, less a product of our genes than of how we take care of ourselves. How well, or how poorly, you age, is in very large part up to you.

What You Can Control

There are five major factors that cause aging. When you understand their impact on every system of the body, you can slow the decline and prolong youthful vitality. No matter how old you are, you'll have more going for you in terms of energy, memory, mobility, keener senses, a fitter body, and more. If you control these factors as they apply to every key system in your body, you'll be postponing old age. Let's talk about the five factors now.

Factor #1: Inflammation: Your Body's Wildfire

Want to prevent heart problems, diabetes, or cancer? How about joint stiffness or dementia? Then pay close attention to what inflammation can do to your body.

Inflammation is essentially a fire within the body that helps to battle germs and responds to trauma and injury. It's normally temporary and beneficial to the healing process. Specifically, inflammation begins when pro-inflammatory hormones dispatch troops of white blood cells to fight infection and repair damaged tissue. Once those threats are over, anti-inflammatory hormones are called in to complete the healing process. This chain of events is referred to as "acute" inflammation. It ebbs and flows within your body and is very important for overall healing. An example is when you're aiming for a nail in the wall but instead you hit your thumbnail with the hammer. The thumb swells and turns red almost immediately; these are signs of normal inflammation—indicators that your immune system is doing its job.

But sometimes that fire rages or gets out of control. What started as a normal, healthy mechanism, doesn't ebb—it keeps flowing. When this occurs in dangerous places, such as your arteries or joints, there is cell damage, and you can become quite ill and debilitated. This type of inflammation is termed "chronic." In fact, it's this kind of inflammation that's thought to be at the core of almost every modern disease known to man, from heart disease to Alzheimer's to cancer. In heart disease, for example, viruses like pneumonia may travel from the lungs to the heart via immune cells, causing chronic inflammation and a diseased heart. In the case of Alzheimer's disease, inflammation triggers the formation of amyloid proteins in the brain. These proteins turn into plaques, disrupting the workings of the brain. Brain plaques are a chief characteristic of Alzheimer's disease. As for cancer, inflammation is the culprit in about 15 percent of all cancers. We don't understand exactly how it does its damage, but scientists believe that inflammation unleashes a type of protein that promotes cellular changes, including the spread of cancer cells.

We don't know exactly what causes chronic inflammation, but we do know that you can actually inflame your body if you smoke, get overweight, never exercise, and can't manage stress. Sound familiar? Pretty much everyone I know has been guilty of something on this list in their lifetime. But it's not too late to extinguish the inflammation in your body, even if you've put your health on the back burner for many years.

Factor #2: Oxidative Stress:
Your Body Is "Rusting"

Have you ever noticed how iron rusts so quickly? The reason for that rust is a chemical process called oxidation, which means electrons are being removed from an atom or molecule in the iron. Now, oxidation itself isn't a bad thing—it goes on around us and in our bodies all the time. But too much oxidation is called oxidative stress, which essentially means the cells in your body are being damaged. Oxidative stress further depletes anti-oxidants, injures tissues, and leaves you vulnerable to premature aging.

Free radicals are the enemy in this situation. By-products of your body's processing of oxygen, free radicals are unstable molecules because each is minus an electron. In other words, while an oxygen atom normally has a nucleus with paired electrons orbiting around it, free radicals have an unpaired electron, so they go around stealing electrons to stabilize themselves. During their quest for an electron, they fire off charges, and those charges damage other cells around them. Thus, the rust.

Over time, free radicals can amass in the body and lead to major health problems, such as cancer, diabetes, atherosclerosis, Alzheimer's disease, and rheumatoid arthritis.

If free radicals are the enemy, then who is your ally in the war against aging? Antioxidants! As you might be able to guess from their name, antioxidants can actually give one of their electrons to the free radicals.

Factor #3: Glycation:
Are You Tangled Up?

"Glycation" sounds like something good, like "vacation's" good friend, don't you think? But no—glycation is a bad thing. It's a process in your body in which the sugar and protein molecules from your food all get stuck together, causing a big, tangled mess. (Imagine your hair on its worst day without conditioner or detangler: no comb can get through that mane.)

So this tough, jumbled tissue mass, as you can imagine, wreaks havoc on the flexibility of your organs, actually causing them to stiffen. Stiffness in, say, your heart can drastically affect its ability to pump blood.

Glycated tissues in your body often produce something aptly named

AGEs, or advanced glycation end-products. These bad guys cause damage throughout your cells and can lead to many age-related diseases including diabetes, Alzheimer's, stroke, and cataracts, and they can even make you look older because they cause wrinkles!

If red blood cells get glycated, they'll have a shortened life span. Your body won't get as much oxygen as it did before, and you'll feel tired, run down, and out of breath frequently. Glycated white blood cells are unable to fight infection, meaning you'll get sick more often. Molecules of LDL cholesterol (the "bad" kind) can become glycated too—a process that prevents the normal shutdown of cholesterol synthesis in the liver. As a result, cholesterol levels soar, increasing the risk of atherosclerosis (hardening of the arteries) and causing cardiac deterioration.

Factor #4: Methylation: Put the Brakes on Aging

If you want to increase your mental capabilities, prevent an untimely death from a heart attack or stroke, and keep cancer far away, you should get familiar with a biological process called methylation. This is a vital process within your body's cells because it determines whether you correctly absorb and properly integrate vitamins, enzymes, and numerous other chemical compounds in the body.

Methylation is directly related to DNA, the molecule that gives your body's cells a "blueprint" on how to function properly. Think of your DNA as little architects creating blueprints for your other cells. Methylation acts like a gas pedal or brake. It can turn unnecessary gene activity up or down and prevents abnormal DNA division so abnormalities aren't passed on to future generations of cells. When it's occurring correctly, methlyation keeps your DNA in good working condition.

Proper methylation can therefore actually slow down aging when it's balanced. However, when methylation is unbalanced, aging speeds up.

The efficiency of methylation in the body naturally declines with age, which is bad news because impaired methylation prevents the production and repair of DNA—a life-threatening situation that can lead to cancer.

So how do you make sure your body is methylating properly, regardless of your age? You can treat the cause, which is often a deficiency in the B vitamin, folic acid. There are foods you can eat such as eggs and seeds that are high in folic acid, and there are medications you can avoid because they cause improper absorption of folic acid. It's really that simple.

Factor #5: Immune Impairment: Don't Let Your Guard Down

One way we get sick is by catching something, such as a cold, a sore throat, or an infection of some type. One of the main reasons we catch something is that our immune system is impaired, and millions of infectious particles invade our body. You've got to keep your immune "guard" at the ready!

Your immune system is pretty much all over your body. Your skin is part of it, your mucous membranes are part of it; many of your organs play an important role in it. And its purpose? To keep you healthy. It is composed of two major parts: the innate immune system and the adaptive immune system. Both undergo changes as we age.

Innate immunity is our first line of defense in the war against infection. I'm talking about your skin, the mucous membranes in your nose, even your stomach acid. Think of these as major obstacles to potential threats. If the germs get past those obstacles, they'll be up against disease-fighting cells like your white blood cells, which will hopefully fight them off.

But as we get older, it seems our innate immune cells don't communicate as well with each other as they once did in our youth. Because of the lack of healthy communication between them, we're more vulnerable to everyday viruses and bacteria. Our "guard" is down.

The adaptive immune system is a bigger network within your body, involving your thymus, spleen, tonsils, bone marrow, circulatory system, and lymphatic system. These organs and systems work in harmony to fight off potential health threats. It's really quite amazing when everything is working at full throttle.

And what if it's not? How can you tell if your immune system isn't working up to par? Easy: if you're getting a lot of colds and flu every year, if it takes sores and infections a long time to heal, or if your white blood cell count is low as indicated through your annual blood work, then your immune system is weakening. You can bolster it easily with regular hand washing, proper nutrition (lots of fruits, veggies, and lean protein, and fewer processed foods), none-to-moderate alcohol intake, and no smoking.

It's worth mentioning here that all five factors of aging are somewhat interrelated, so the lifestyle and behavior changes you make in one factor impact the other four. My general recommendations that follow will make a significant and lasting impact on every system of the body, and ultimately your health and longevity. Here are my general recommendations for controlling each of the five factors of aging:

My Recommendations to Stop and Prevent Inflammation

Get into a healthy weight range. Because being above the range of healthy weight for your height has been identified as a major trigger for inflammation, you'll find that I encourage you to take steps toward weight loss in conjunction with all of my other anti-aging recommendations. And I have great news: studies show that the more weight you lose, the more your C-reactive protein (CRP) levels will drop. Don't confuse that with CPR. By CRP, I'm talking about a protein that can be detected in the blood as part of your annual routine blood tests. This protein indicates how much inflammation is going on in your body. But back to weight loss and inflammation: With each pound lost, just imagine water being dumped on the flames of inflammation in your body.

Move yourself. Exercise is a vital component in keeping your weight down, plus it seems to relieve inflammation as well. If you exercise more than 22 times a month, you can reduce your CRP levels significantly, according to a study from Emory University School of Medicine. You'll hear me say this a lot: healthy exercise means a healthy body now and for decades ahead. Exercise can mean anything from a 30-minute walk to weight training to fast-dancing the night away . . . so get movin'!

Know your fat facts. Eat good fats, and you'll prevent or reduce inflammation. Fish is loaded with good fats (omega-3 fatty acids), and these fats have been linked to lower inflammation and less arthritis pain in some clinical studies. Extra-virgin olive oil also has some great anti-inflammatory properties. So do walnuts and flaxseeds.

Enjoy good carbs. Foods like whole grains, fruits, vegetables, and beans are abundant in good carbs and are super rich in fiber, which is an inflammation fighter. University of Massachusetts researchers found that people who ate the most fiber had the lowest CRP levels. Refined carbohydrates (sweets, processed foods, or commercially baked foods) have the opposite effect; they are inflammation magnets. So avoid white bread, sugar, low-fiber cereals, and most man-made carbs. They stoke the inflammation fires in your body.

Rethink your drink. Milk has gotten a bad rap in a lot of circles, but guess what? It's an effective anti-inflammatory. That's because it's a top source of vitamin D, which can quell inflammation. Low levels of D in the blood have been linked to both osteoarthritis and rheumatoid arthritis, two diseases with inflammation as the culprit. Sunshine and multivitamins also provide D. Alcoholic beverages, in moderation, may also ease inflammation. Moderation means one drink a day. More than that, and you risk fanning the flames of inflammation.

My Recommendations to Stop and Prevent Oxidative Stress

Take supplemental antioxidants. Vitamins A, C, E, and beta-carotene all provide antioxidants, as do selenium, bioflavonoids, and the herbs ginkgo biloba and ginseng. Your local health food store or pharmacy should have a wide selection of antioxidant multivitamin and mineral formulations in stock for you to choose from.

Eat colorful, antioxidant-rich foods. Colorful fruits and vegetables contain antioxidants known as carotenoids, which are the phytonutrients that give fruits and vegetables their distinctive yellow, orange, and red colors.

Choose green. Green foods such as barley grass, green tea, and any green leafy vegetable are loaded with life-extending antioxidants for optimal inner health, immune support, and a high level of well-being.

Exercise at the right level. Exercise, when you're doing it correctly, raises your antioxidant levels faster than free radicals can be produced. But if you overdo exercise, you can actually increase inflammation. How do you know if you've overdone it? Symptoms including swelling, unusual fatigue, or muscle soreness that doesn't dissipate after 48 hours.

My Recommendations to Stop and Prevent Glycation

Say no to high fructose corn syrup (HFCS). This is a particularly nasty form of refined sugar, used widely as an additive in many processed foods such as soft drinks, breakfast cereals, candy, and chips. My advice is to find the hidden sugars in your diet (read labels; any substance ending in "ose" is an added sugar) and limit your sugar intake altogether, if you want to look and feel young.

Eat blueberries. Blueberries are packed with anti-inflammatory pigments called anthocyanins that give them their deep blue color. Scientific studies have revealed that anthocyanins naturally avert glycation by fortifying the collagen in your skin and improving microcirculation (pumped-up circulation via capillaries). Eat more blueberries (in smoothies, on cereals, or just plain), and your skin will start looking more youthful. Eat up!

Supplement against glycation. There are a number of supplements you can take that protect against destructive glycation reactions: carnosine, an amino acid compound found primarily in red meat that protects the heart and brain cells from glycation; pyridoxal-5-phosphate, the active form of vitamin B-6; and benfotiamine, a fat-soluble form of thiamine (vitamin B-1).

My Recommendations to Balance Methylation

Eat some eggs. Egg yolks contain high levels of vitamin B-12 and folic acid, both of which are key in ensuring balance in your cells' methylation. Eggs have been vilified for their cholesterol content for years, but new research indicates that their nutritional benefits outweigh their risks. This isn't a green light to chow down on a three-egg omelet every morning; one yolk and a couple of whites should do the trick. Alternatively or in conjunction, take vitamin B-12 oral supplements.

Check your meds. Even if you're chasing your morning medications with handfuls of multivitamins or supplements, certain medications interfere drastically with your body's absorption of vitamins, including B-12, perhaps the most important vitamin in balancing methylation. If you're regularly taking acid blockers for reflux, you could be absorbing as little as one-quarter of the B-12 you're eating. Talk to your doctor about B-12 supplements, of which there are many forms such as oral or sublingual, if your levels are low.

Snack on seeds. Sunflower seeds pack a major nutritional punch because they're loaded with folic acid (the mighty methylation regulator), thiamin, niacin . . . the list goes on. Munch on a few as a snack, or sprinkle a tablespoon on a salad or in soup. Same goes for pumpkin seeds, chia seeds, and sesame seeds. But watch for sodium here; grab the unsalted kind. And they're more caloric than you'd think, so don't overdo.

My Recommendations to Stop and Prevent Immune Impairment

Wash your paws! Believe it or not, hand washing is still the first line of defense when it comes to bacterial or viral invaders. Good old-fashioned soap and water is the single most important factor in preventing infection and keeping your immune system strong and safe. So, suds up for at least 20 seconds several times a day, especially before eating and after visiting the bathroom.

Get your shots. Vaccines you should consider include adult tetanus shots (required every 10 years—sooner if there is a dirty wound) and possibly others, including Pneumovax to prevent pneumonia, flu shots, and hepatitis vaccines. Talk to your doctor about which immunizations are appropriate for you.

Pump up your nutrition. Slight deficiencies in zinc, copper, selenium, and/or vitamins A, C, E, B-6, D, and folic acid can zap your immune system. Avert deficiencies by choosing nutrient-dense foods and supplementing with a good multivitamin-mineral antioxidant.

Quit smoking. This is one of the anti-aging essentials, which are the five things I want you start working on immediately; you'll find them in the next chapter. It goes without saying that quitting smoking will rid your body of the toxins in cigarettes. After a few hours of quitting, the high amounts of nicotine and carbon monoxide in your system begin to normalize. Within a month of quitting, your risks of lung infection decrease, as well as your blood pressure. Ten years after quitting, your immune system is recharged, and your risk of cancer can drop by 30 to 50 percent.

Use antibiotics only for bacterial infections. You'd be surprised by how many of my patients call me up with a simple cold and instruct me to prescribe antibiotics. Okay, people, here's the truth. Antibiotics treat only bacterial infections, which have to be diagnosed. Why does it matter if you take them for something else? It matters because of a little something called antibiotic resistance. This means that if you abuse them when you *don't* need them, they can't work for you when you *do*. Antibiotic resistance is a huge problem, perhaps one of the largest (and scariest) health issues threatening our world today.

When you take antibiotics, your body produces fewer cytokines, the hormone messengers of the immune system. This, in turn, suppresses your immune system, meaning you're more susceptible to resistant bacteria. Here's a short list of the illnesses getting harder to treat: pneumonia, sinus infections, skin infections, and tuberculosis. Trust me, you don't want any these illnesses, nor do you want to live in a society where everyone else has them because they've become resistant to antibiotics.

So take antibiotics *only* for bacterial infections, use them right away, and take the entire prescription. Don't use antibiotics preventively unless your doctor advises it.

The path to living 100 happy, healthy years does not begin with and may not ever run through the CCUs, ICUs, clinics, ORs, and ERs where medical care is rendered. True vitality and longevity come about by focusing on lifestyle strategies that will keep you out of such places to begin with. But in order to change, you have to know the reasons and ways these strategies de-age. Knowledge truly is power. The more you know, the better you can take care of yourself, and the longer you can live happily and productively. We've simply got to move in that direction, and I'm here to show you how. If you can control any of these five factors of aging—and you can—then, congratulations, you're on your way to living 100 happy, healthy years.

CHAPTER 2

Build Your Anti-Aging Base

I f you were building a house, where would you start? The foundation, right? You can't exactly install flooring and put up wallpaper without a strong, solid base to support the structure. Think of this chapter as building the foundation for your soon-to-be newly fortified body. That foundation is made up of five basic building blocks that support every one of your body's systems in unique and often surprising ways.

These elements are movement (yes, I mean exercise, and I know some people think of this as a dirty word, but I'm not just talking about the kind where you go the gym and sweat it out on the treadmill), avoiding smoking of any kind (cigarette, cigar, pipe, etc.), maintaining a healthy weight (I'll show you how to figure out what "healthy" means for your body), staying hydrated, and taking the right supplements. These basic, essential elements are my first five anti-aging essentials.

You'll find these mentioned again in my system-specific chapters so I can show you exactly how they have a distinct effect on each of your systems; this way, you can really *understand* why you're following these prescriptions. I can sit here all day long and give you a laundry list of overall do's and don'ts for preserving your health. But first, that's a pretty boring book, and second, I know from experience that patients aren't willing to commit to recommendations of any kind unless they understand why they're following them. For example, you may realize that exercise improves your circulation, but did you know it can also improve your sex life because of its positive effects on your reproductive system? (Yes, I'll be pulling out all the stops in an effort to get you moving!)

So, you may think you know why these anti-aging basics are important, but by the time you've finished this book, you'll have a whole new understanding. In just 17 days, if you follow my simple plan, you'll likely have more energy, look rejuvenated, and weigh less, and you'll have taken major strides toward increasing your life expectancy.

Without further ado, let's begin building your foundation, shall we?

#1: Movement

Think you need an expensive gym membership in order to make exercise a priority in your life? Unless you're surrounded by sweaty, bodybuilding dudes pumping iron and high-ponytailed women donning spandex while prancing on the treadmill, then you couldn't possibly be taking exercise seriously, right? Wrong. So many people have the wrong idea in their heads that burning calories and building muscles are actions that can only occur within the confines of a gym. That is categorically untrue. It doesn't matter whether you're trudging your way through a half hour on the Stairmaster or walking up the stairs instead of taking the elevator in your office building . . . you're still torching calories, incinerating fat, and increasing your muscle mass. Your body doesn't know or care whether you take it to a fancy sports club with state-of-the-art equipment or if you are just taking an extra lap around the block before you walk into a store; it is going to experience the positive effects of your decision to get moving regardless of where, when, or how you move.

This idea was so intriguing to researchers at the Mayo Clinic that they did a study to prove that it works, and they gave it a name: NEAT, which stands for nonexercise activity thermogenesis. NEAT refers to all the things you do when you aren't purposely exercising: pacing while on the phone, walking somewhere instead of hopping in the car, climbing stairs, cleaning the house . . . and the list goes on. In the study, volunteers consumed 1,000 calories more per day than their bodies needed. The participants who consistently engaged in NEAT burned off much more of those excess calories than the subjects who didn't, and thus gained less fat over the study period. Imagine what would happen if you didn't overeat and you increased your NEAT. You can burn hundreds, even thousands, of extra calories just by finding little ways to move more every day.

Right now, today, I'd like you to start finding all kinds of ways to move—from the moment you wake up until the moment you go to bed. Pace around the bathroom while you brush your teeth (what else could you possibly have to do then?), park farther away from the entrance to the grocery store so you have to walk and carry your bags, go on a stroll during your lunch break, stand up to fold the laundry (and maybe do some squats while you fold!)—there are endless ways to move more, folks. You don't even have to be all that creative to come up with them! If it helps, write a few down and post them somewhere that you'll see. Better yet, put them in your online calendar so it will send you a reminder. Do whatever it takes, but increase your movement today, and you've just taken your very first and very important step on the path to anti-aging your entire body. Not to mention the fact that you're going to look really good, too!

#2: Maintain a Healthy Weight

First, here are what I consider to be healthy weight ranges for men and women, based on height. There are exceptions, and I will get to those, but for the vast majority of people, these numbers are accurate. The weight smack in the middle of these ranges is the one I want you to aim for.

WOMEN			
4'10"	81	**90**	99
4'11"	86	**95**	105
5'	90	**100**	110
5'1"	95	**105**	116
5'2"	99	**110**	121
5'3"	104	**115**	127
5'4"	108	**120**	132
5'5"	113	**125**	138
5'6"	117	**130**	143
5'7"	122	**135**	149
5'8"	126	**140**	154
5'9"	131	**145**	160
5'10"	135	**150**	165
5'11"	140	**155**	171
6'	144	**160**	176
6'1"	149	**165**	182
6'2"	153	**170**	187

MEN			
5'3"	112	**124**	136
5'4"	117	**130**	143
5'5"	122	**136**	150
5'6"	128	**142**	156
5'7"	133	**148**	163
5'8"	139	**154**	169
5'9"	144	**161**	176
5'10"	149	**166**	183
5'11"	155	**172**	189
6'	160	**178**	196
6'1"	166	**184**	202
6'2"	171	**190**	209
6'3"	176	**196**	216
6'4"	182	**202**	222
6'5"	187	**208**	229
6'6"	193	**214**	235
6'7"	198	**220**	242

If you are already at a healthy weight, let me congratulate you and encourage you to maintain it. If you aren't, let me empower you to target your healthy weight and, using my tools, reach it.

I mentioned exceptions: If you are any kind of extreme athlete (body-builder, Olympic swimmer, ultra-marathoner), your weight may differ from the ranges listed above. But if you say, "That weight range is impossible for me because I am big-boned and so is my entire family," then you are not an exception; you simply fall in the higher end of the healthy range for your height. And that's fine! Not everyone has to hit that middle number on their scale. You simply need to change your outlook and start applying the techniques I discuss in *The 17 Day Diet*. For instance, some of the first steps I recommend in Cycle 1 of *The 17 Day Diet* are to reduce your carbohydrate intake (especially sugar, sweets, and refined carbohydrates), increase your protein intake (especially lean meats), drink more water, and add more veggies (especially green ones) to your plate.

Getting yourself into a healthy weight range and maintaining those habits so the needle on the scale doesn't move much is a huge part of controlling the five factors of aging. This is especially true when it comes to inflammation, which we know is triggered by excess weight. The benefits spread across all of your body's systems, sometimes in shocking ways, which I'll discuss in later chapters. Here's just one example to get you going: *The Journal of the American Medical Association* reported on a study involving 48 overweight people. They cut their calories by 25 percent over several months, and some pretty fascinating things started happening in their bodies. Of course they lost weight, but researchers found that these test subjects also had a drop in their insulin levels. This cut their risk for serious illnesses like type 2 diabetes and heart disease. But there was more: They also showed a decrease in the amount of DNA damage occurring throughout their body, meaning their organs were experiencing less oxidative stress. Less oxidative stress means a lower production of free radicals, which means a reduced risk of Alzheimer's disease, coronary artery disease, Parkinson's disease, and much more. Reducing your caloric intake by 25 percent if you are overweight is a very small commitment when you compare it to the incredible anti-aging rewards it provides to your body and all its systems.

#3: Stay Hydrated

It never ceases to amaze me how many people walk (or run!) around all day long—working, taking care of kids, running errands, exercising, or even just hanging out—completely ignorant of the fact that every cell in their body is desperate for water. Maybe you think that cup of coffee at 8 a.m. and few sips of a diet soda with lunch are enough to keep you going, especially if you aren't dying of thirst. I have so many patients that come in complaining of vertigo, or dizziness, and very often they've been experiencing it for weeks. They expect me to talk to them about all kinds of serious illnesses that cause dizziness and prescribe some medication to make it subside, so they're usually a little taken aback when I hand them a sheet from my prescription pad that says, "Drink more water!"

If you are not drinking six to eight glasses of water per day, or more if you're on your feet a lot or exercising regularly, you are not drinking enough water. Maybe you're like many of my patients who say you just hate water and would rather drink coffee, soda, or juice. Then it's a good thing you're reading this book, because I'm going to give you all kinds of ways to learn to love water. I'm also going to help you understand, system by system, why your body is craving it more than you realize . . . but even more exciting . . . I'm going to show you how the simple act of hydration can work wonders to prevent so many signs of aging. There are really surprising ways that water can work magic in your body—from keeping the mucous lining of your lungs robust, thus improving your breathing, to boosting your memory and regulating digestion. I'm really passionate about getting people to increase their water intake. Maybe that seems silly to you, but just try it and I'll make you a believer in good, old-fashioned H_2O!

#4: Avoid Smoking

You are not exempt from reading this section just because you don't light up the moment you get in the car, take cigarette breaks, blow through a pack a day, or smoke cigars after dinner. I am also talking to those of you who occasionally or "socially" smoke cigarettes, cigars, pipes, joints, and so forth, as well as those of you who use chewing tobacco or suck in secondhand smoke on a regular basis. But don't worry; this won't feel like you're watching one of those terrifying antismoking public service announcements. Do I want you to quit? Of course. Do I think you need to be scared silly in order to do so? Absolutely not. But a healthy dose of logic goes a long way in this area.

I happen to believe that most smokers, even social smokers, have something similar to a split personality. Now, I'm not diagnosing all smokers with schizophrenia! I'm simply referring to the two voices you likely have in your head. One is your logical side, the voice that says, "You know this isn't good for you. You don't even feel all that great doing it. You've heard it can cause cancer—heck, even the pack of cigarettes has photos of decaying lungs on it. You should really quit. After this one." And then your smoker side says, "What? It's not like I'm doing drugs or something. There are lots of people that smoke way more than me—and they're just fine! I just don't want to go through the withdrawals, gain all that weight, and turn into a total moody freak. I'll wait until I can get through this month and then try quitting. Again." Is that pretty close to your internal dispute? Perhaps the excuses differ somewhat, but this is the story many smokers have told me.

Right now, allow me to directly address the smoker voice in your head. You are a thief. You are stealing away minutes, hours, days, months, years from your own future. Here's the worst part: You are not your only victim. Every time you put a cigarette to your lips, you are committing a crime against your family and your friends who love and need you both now and later in life. Even if you do live for a long time, odds are very good that if you continue smoking, even occasionally, your body will incur damage and you won't be the healthiest, happiest version of yourself as you get older.

Anyone who wants to live 100 happy, healthy years can't keep smoking. It's that simple. They are mutually exclusive, period. And if you think I'm just talking about the effects smoking has on your lungs, prepare yourself, because I'm going to show you the effects smoking has on every system and organ in your body, from your brain to your hormones, bone density, kidneys, reproductive system . . . all of it.

#5: Supplements

I'm never going to tell you to just pop a pill as a way to get healthier or stop the effects of aging. Too many folks think they can make up for a multitude of nutritional bloopers by popping fistfuls of vitamins, minerals, and supplements. For instance, if you're a sworn veggie-hater (and I *will* convert you; by the way, whose idea of lean meat is a single-patty burger instead of double?), a chewable multivitamin every morning will not cover your bases.

Here's the deal: I want you to get most of your essential nutrients, which include vitamins and minerals, from the foods that you're eating. I feel that synthetic supplements will never be as good as the real thing. Given a choice, I will always guide you toward the most natural solutions, and vitamins are in their most natural form within foods. However, you'll find system-specific supplement recommendations in each section of this book. That's because, all too often, it can be difficult to come by the freshest, most nutrient-dense foods, and I want you to have an understanding of which nutrients will support which systems and functions the most. I think that you'll be more likely to find ways to consume these nutrients if you understand why they're good for you to begin with. If you know that you need an extra boost in certain body systems, you'll find the targeted supplements that will help within those chapters.

You will read a lot about antioxidants like beta-carotene and vitamin C in this book, and you'll marvel at the wonders these can work to anti-age essentially all of your systems. So, my prescription is to start eating fruits and vegetables in addition to taking that multivitamin every morning. But there's more you can do to target each of your systems and to ensure that you're getting the nutrients that will work the hardest for you.

So, there you have them: No matter which system you're targeting, these essential elements are going to be at the core of your new, reinforced body that could last you 100 years and beyond. Now follow me on a journey into each of your body's incredible systems so I can show you my strategies for fortifying every one of them against the battering rams of time. You're well on your way to 100 healthy, happy years.

PART TWO

* *

Cycle 1: Restore

You might consider the heart, lungs, and brain as solitary parts of the circulatory, respiratory, and neurological systems, but all three affect and are affected by virtually all parts of the body. Chronic lung diseases, such as emphysema, can abnormally enlarge the heart and affect blood pressure, for example. Mild kidney disease increases the chance of a heart attack or stroke. Endocrine problems involving insulin and glucose abnormalities associated with diabetes can lead to disease of the small blood vessels in the brain, causing dementia. What's more, depression, anxiety, and chronic stress can promote heart disease or make it worse. High blood pressure, cholesterol-clogged arteries, inflammation, and other risk factors for heart disease are implicated in Alzheimer's disease.

I could go on and on here, but I want to get you right into Cycle 1: Restore, in which we revitalize these three interconnected systems. Preventing problems in these systems is a prerequisite to ensuring health and longevity.

So let's roll right into Cycle 1. You're about to discover what I consider to be the most effective things you can do for restoring these three systems, the best strategies for creating health and longevity, and the best plan I can think of for staying out of the doctor's office.

CHAPTER 3

The Heart of the Matter

What if you could avoid having a heart attack? That's right; I'm asking if you'd do what was needed to avoid the story we've all heard before—the horrifying experience of having a searing, stabbing pain in your chest that spreads to your arms, neck, or jaw, and that moment when the brutal realization sets in that your life is in jeopardy. I'm not saying avoiding this scenario is as simple for everyone as following my prescription, but we do know that it's possible to prevent up to 80 percent of heart disease diagnoses in this country.

Every year, 1.25 million Americans suffer a heart attack, and it frustrates me to no end; as a doctor, I know so many causes of heart disease are preventable and even reversible. And I'm not necessarily talking about pharmaceuticals as the solution. I'm just as amazed by how far we've come with our treatment options (surgery, outpatient procedures, and prescription drugs) as anyone else. But when you really think about it, much of "modern medicine" is about slowing down a disease that's already got a hold on you. It's about treatment, and what I'm talking about here is actually prevention of disease and preservation of good health.

Heart attack, angina (chest pain), stroke, high blood pressure, high cholesterol, and the buildup of plaque on the vessel walls known as atherosclerosis are serious, often life-threatening conditions that affect your circulatory system. Think of the people you know who have had a heart attack. Now think about eliminating that suffering for eight out of 10 of them, and eight out of 10 of their families. It can be done!

Circulatory System 101

I'm the kind of the doctor who believes in educating patients as a part of healing, so pardon me while I launch into a little Circulatory System 101.

Your body has *two* circulatory systems: One sends blood from the heart to the lungs and back (this is called pulmonary circulation) and the other sends blood from the heart to the rest of the body (this is systemic circulation).

Every day, your circulatory system transports blood to your body's tissues, carrying oxygen and nutrients to every single cell. It pumps the 10 pints of blood in your body through your 60,000 miles of blood vessels that link the cells of our organs and body parts.

The Heart

The heart rules the circulatory system. Some fascinating statistics: Your heart beats about 100,000 times a day, more than 30 million times per year, and about 2.5 billion times over an average lifetime. Your brain sends messages to the heart, telling it when to pump more or less blood, depending on your needs and what you're doing. When you're asleep, it pumps just enough to provide for the lower amounts of oxygen needed by your body at rest. When you're exercising or scared, the heart pumps more rapidly to get more oxygen to power your muscles.

The Role of Blood Vessels

You have three different types of blood vessels. First, you have arteries, which carry blood away from your heart. They are the thickest blood vessels, thanks to their muscular walls that contract to maintain blood flow. In the systemic circulation, oxygen-rich blood is pumped from the heart into the aorta, the large artery that curves up and back from the heart. Two coronary arteries crown the heart, branch off at the beginning of the aorta, and divide into branches of smaller arteries that oxygenate and nourish heart muscles.

The second type of blood vessels are veins. They carry blood back to the heart and have tiny valves that keep the blood flowing in the correct direction.

Finally, you have tiny capillaries, which connect the arteries and veins. They deliver nutrients and oxygen to your cells. They're like little trash men who work just for you, because they're also responsible for removing waste products such as carbon dioxide from the body.

Your whole body depends on the work your circulatory system does, and it's very much interconnected with all of your other systems. It's like a giant network of highways and roads, transporting vital nutrients and hormones to where they need to go.

How Your Circulatory System Ages

Not long ago, doctors viewed heart disease as the by-product of clogged blood vessels. Cholesterol levels in the blood go up, and, over the years, these fatty deposits clog the pipes and cut off the blood supply, or break off and create clots. But we've since come to better understand cholesterol and its role in our bodies.

Everyone thinks of cholesterol as a bad word. You may be surprised to learn that cholesterol is actually essential to your body's overall health. And get this . . . cholesterol plays an integral role in your body's production of hormones. I'll bet you didn't know that!

Sixty to 80 percent of your cholesterol is carried by low-density lipoproteins (LDL), which are molecular "postmen" that deliver cholesterol from the liver to cells to build cell membranes. Unfortunately, the cells don't usually need all the cholesterol that's delivered; the excess cholesterol is like junk mail that piles up as plaque on artery walls and can lead to atherosclerosis. That's why LDL is what we call "bad" cholesterol. Twenty to 40 percent of your cholesterol is ferried by high-density lipoproteins (HDL), known as "good" cholesterol because it roams the bloodstream, scavenging bits of bad cholesterol and carrying them back to the liver for disposal.

A little trick I use to differentiate "good" from "bad" cholesterol is to think of the "L" versus the "H." LDL can be thought to stand for "lousy," so it should be low. HDL can stand for "happy," so it should be high. It's good to understand the difference so you're prepared when your doctor tells you about your numbers or in case you perform at-home cholesterol testing, which I do recommend for folks who need to closely monitor their cholesterol or for folks who don't have insurance.

About 85 percent of the cholesterol your body needs is produced by your liver. Another 15 percent comes from the food you eat. Normally, your body maintains an equilibrium in regard to how much cholesterol it requires. If you eat too many high-cholesterol foods, your liver will compensate by making less cholesterol. That's the best-case scenario, but of course it's not always the case; what can really jack up your cholesterol is eating a lot of saturated fat from animal fats and protein. This causes fat to build up in your arteries and other blood vessels.

At the turn of the 20th century, scientists had a strong suspicion that cholesterol played a role in heart disease because they found that when people died of heart attacks, some or a lot of cholesterol could always be detected in their arteries. But cholesterol didn't become public enemy number one until the 1950s and '60s, when deaths from heart attacks skyrocketed in the United States.

Cholesterol is not the only risk factor for heart disease. Strange but true, now we know that nearly 50 percent of all heart attacks occur in people with normal cholesterol levels and normal blood pressure. Something causes relatively minor deposits to burst, triggering massive clots that block the blood supply.

That "something" has turned out to be inflammation.

C-reactive protein (CRP) is a blood measure of inflammation. Research has revealed that those with the highest CRP levels have three times the heart attack risk as those with the lowest levels.

That's because inflammation ages your heart muscle. It puts your most precious muscle under stress and makes it work harder to pump blood than it did when you were younger. Plus, inflammation can cause your blood vessels to get less flexible and fatty deposits to collect on the inner walls of your arteries (atherosclerosis). These changes stiffen your arteries. As the arteries stiffen (or harden), your heart has to work overtime in order to get blood through them. And that, my friends, is what very often leads to something I hate to see in patients: high blood pressure (hypertension).

Lifestyle choices such as not exercising, eating too much salt, drinking too much alcohol, and eating too much junk food will often lead to high blood pressure. The higher your blood pressure is over time, the shorter your life expectancy. Although high blood pressure is a "silent disease," there can definitely be symptoms, such as vision problems, breathlessness, and nosebleeds. In addition to seeing your doctor for regular checkups, which will include taking your blood pressure, watch carefully for those symptoms and don't hesitate to alert your doctor if you experience them.

If you have high cholesterol, and lifestyle changes haven't helped, talk to your doc about statins. You may have heard about the ability of statins to lower cholesterol, but the recent research shows that statin drugs may also have anti-inflammatory properties. Studies indicate that statins can reduce blood levels of CRP, that key marker for inflammation. Find out from your physician if you're a good candidate for these drugs. (Keep in mind that these drugs come with a slew of potential side effects including muscle aches, headaches, nausea, weakness, upset stomach, and joint pain. I see these problems all the time.) In the box on supplements that support your circulatory system in this chapter, you'll find a list of over-the-counter supplements I tell my patients who cannot tolerate statins to try.

A healthy circulatory system, in good working order, is essential to living 100 healthy years. As with so many aspects of our health, we take it for granted until complications arise. If you have high blood pressure, you are at an increased risk of having a stroke. You're also in a higher risk category of having a heart attack. Did you catch that? Let me reiterate: High blood pressure means you are more likely to have a heart attack. Think that's it? Nope. High blood pressure, over time, can also take you down the road to kidney failure and damage to your vision. That needs to stop—right now. Take care of your circulatory system *before* trouble starts.

Top Strategies for a Healthy Heart
Nutrition

As a family practice physician, I spend a lot of time counseling patients about diet and nutrition. Nutritional strategies will prevent your circulatory system from aging if you follow an anti-inflammatory diet. Yes, there are foods that will help put out the fires of inflammation that might be raging in your body and slow down the aging process. Isn't it astounding that just putting the right foods in your mouth could actually save your life? I know it seems basic, but so many people miss this. If you are hoping to make it to the century mark like I am, I suggest you eat more of the following anti-inflammatory foods:

Salmon. It's high in omega-3 fatty acids, which reduce inflammation. The best choice is wild-caught salmon. (Avoid farm-raised salmon; it's higher in arachidonic acid, as well as toxins, all of which increase inflammation.) Herring, mackerel, and sardines are also loaded with omega-3s.

Walnuts. These nuts are another plentiful source of omega-3s and other healthful compounds, including vitamin E, which is a powerful immune booster.

Onions. Onions are rich in quercetin, a type of antioxidant that prevents harmful enzymes from triggering inflammation. Onions also contain sulfur compounds that bolster the immune system. Other good sources of quercetin include apples, broccoli, red wine, red grapes, grape juice, and tea.

Blueberries. I can't say enough great things about blueberries. Blueberries are packed with anthocyanins, a type of antioxidant that boosts immunity and protects the body from free radical damage (an inflammation trigger). Other good sources of anthocyanins include blackberries, strawberries, raspberries, and cranberries.

Sweet potatoes. Sweet potatoes are rich in carotenoids, a type of antioxidant known for boosting immunity and preventing inflammation. Not a sweet-potato kind of guy or gal? Try chomping down on other orange, red, yellow, or green fruits and veggies like carrots, yellow squash, peppers, and mangoes.

Spinach. Spinach also has carotenoids, not to mention immune-boosting vitamin E. Any green leafy vegetable is powerful for immune support.

Garlic. Like onions, garlic is rich in sulfur compounds that boost the activity of immune cells. Garlic is also a powerful anti-inflammatory agent.

Pineapple. Bromelain, found in pineapple, is an enzyme that decreases inflammation and confers some immune-enhancing effects. Pineapple is also an excellent source of the antioxidant vitamin C.

Ginger. Fresh ginger root acts as an anti-inflammatory. It works by dampening the action of inflammation-promoting enzymes in the body.

Turmeric. The key component in curry, turmeric contains curcumin, a compound that has anti-inflammatory effects.

Pomegranate and pomegranate juice. Revered since ancient times, the pomegranate has recently become acclaimed for its cardiovascular health benefits. It is a powerful antioxidant that appears to protect the heart and blood vessels. Pomegranate juice may have anti-clogging properties, slowing the progression of arterial plaques. It may even reduce blood pressure.

Any and all vegetables. Besides the veggies I mentioned above, I want to emphasize the importance of all vegetables for circulatory health. Vegetables, which many people now refer to as "plant foods," contain phytonutrients—protective disease-fighting substances in foods. Some of these may help the body produce nitric oxide, which is a vasodilator and can help reduce blood pressure. A study published in the July 2011 issue of the *American Journal of Clinical Nutrition* has linked diets rich in vegetables and fruits to better cardiovascular health and overall longevity. Basically, this study looked at total vegetable intake, total fruit intake, and cruciferous vegetable intake in two large groups of Chinese subjects and found that high intakes of total vegetables, particularly the cruciferous ones (such as broccoli, cauliflower, and cabbage), were associated with a significantly reduced risk of death due to cardiovascular disease. Cruciferous vegetables are rich sources of compounds called sulforaphanes, which act as antioxidants and anti-inflammatories in the body. These two effects are of particular importance with respect to heart disease.

CALLING ALL VEGGIE HATERS!

If the thought of a spinach salad makes your stomach turn and you think you wouldn't nosh on a carrot stick if it were the last morsel of food left on Earth, you are, indeed, setting yourself up for some majorly unattractive effects of aging. So, listen up.

There are lots of different vegetables you can eat, not just the ones that offend you the most. Plus, there are thousands of herbs and spices you can add to veggies and endless ways to prepare them, including baking, steaming, grilling, boiling, and hiding them in spaghetti sauce. (Note: You'll find some delicious veggie ideas in the Appendix.) But for goodness' sake, give them a try! If you cut out vegetables from your diet, you're giving up truly key nutrients that your body is craving, even if you aren't listening.

Try this experiment: Trade out one "bad" food (that daily bag of potato chips or slices of white bread) for one veggie every day during Cycle 1. I'm willing to bet you will lose weight. Why? When you're eating vegetables, you're able to eat until you're full without taking in nearly the same number of calories as if you were snacking on processed foods and other unhealthy options.

One study at Tufts University revealed that people who ate the widest variety of vegetables had the least amount of body fat. Live longer and be thinner just munching on a few vegetables a day? Who could refuse that? Put a little effort into learning to love veggies the way anyone who makes it to happy, healthy old age likely does. I dare you!

While there are a ton of terrific foods and recipes that you can add to your diet for strong circulatory health, I would be remiss if I didn't tell you about a few things that can actually promote inflammation in your body, including your circulatory system. These foods hike levels of endothelin, a compound that promotes inflammation in blood vessels, and ultimately, clogging. I've got a long list of foods for you that promote inflammation in your body. Needless to say, you'll want to cut way back on these.

My list starts with foods high in simple sugars. They are directly linked to the development of inflammation in the body and they aggravate the symptoms of inflammation.

Cut back on

White rice
White bread
Packaged snack foods like pretzels, potato chips, and popcorn
White flour
Corn syrups
Regular pasta made with white flour
Sweetened cereals
Pastries such as cakes, donuts, muffins, and pies
Fast food
Sugary sodas
Jams, jellies, and preserves
Alcoholic beverages, especially beer

You should also avoid foods high in LDL cholesterol, trans fats, and saturated fats; they can increase your risk of inflammation. No-no's include the following:

Cut back on

    Butter
    Fried and canned meats
    Pork bacon
    Cocoa butter
    Cream cheese
    Whole milk and other full-fat dairy products
    Corn oil
    Cottonseed oil
    Margarine, shortening, lard, and hydrogenated oils
    Organ meats, such as liver

In my day-to-day work life, I advise patients to watch what they eat as a way to lower inflammation and LDL cholesterol in their bodies. This can be tricky, because not all bodies respond the same way: While some patients make these dietary adjustments and enjoy the benefits of low-ered inflammation and cholesterol, others make a valiant effort to change their junk-food ways but still see no major improvements. Fortunately, there are other strategies, in addition to diet, that you can follow on your journey.

SUPPLEMENTS THAT SUPPORT YOUR CIRCULATORY SYSTEM

If you have high cholesterol and you cannot tolerate statins because of the various side effects they can cause, then I usually recommend a combination of supplements to help you lower your cholesterol without the prescription pad. However, it's imperative that you run it by your own doctor before self-medicating with these supplements.

FOR HIGH-CHOLESTEROL PATIENTS ONLY

- **Niacin:** 250 milligrams a day for two or more weeks until they experience no flushing, which is a common side effect of niacin. After two weeks, I increase their dose to 500 milligrams a day. Once they tolerate that dose well, I increase the dose again to 750 milligrams daily.
- **Fish oil:** 3 grams a day
- **Flaxseed oil:** 1 tablespoon a day (this can be part of a salad dressing)
- **L-carnitine:** 500 milligrams twice daily

- **Coenzyme Q10:** 50 milligrams twice daily
- **Vitamin C:** 1,000 milligrams a day, either buffered (calcium ascorbate) or unbuffered (ascorbic acid)

If you do *not* have high cholesterol, you should still take the following supplements from the above list to support overall function of your circulatory system:

- **Vitamin C:** 1,000 milligrams
- **Flaxseed oil:** 1 tablespoon
- **Coenzyme Q10:** 50 milligrams

REASONS

Niacin is a type of Vitamin B and it can increase your HDL, or good cholesterol. Fish oil can lower your triglycerides and decrease inflammation. Flaxseed oil can boost your HDL. The amino acid L-carnitine can reduce your LDL, or bad cholesterol, and can strengthen heart muscle. Coenzyme Q10 helps deliver more oxygen to the circulatory tissues. Vitamin C helps prevent blood clots.

The Anti-Aging Essentials and Your Circulatory System

#1: Movement. How does exercise affect your heart and circulation? Studies have shown that your body produces fewer inflammatory chemicals if you're physically fit. And how do you get physically fit? Regular cardiovascular exercise is my answer. Engaging in cardiovascular exercise is a powerful way to reduce CRP levels and abdominal fat, not to mention that it helps you get in better shape. Doing cardio might involve walking, jogging, biking, swimming, or taking an aerobic dance class, to name just a few options. If you're not currently active, aim to build up to at least 30 to 45 minutes of exercise three or more days a week. Make it moderate activity. That means you should be breathing more heavily than normal and feel slightly warmer. I also recommend getting into your *cardio zone*, which is 60 to 80 percent of your maximum heart rate for 30 minutes each day. You'll find the formula for this in the Appendix. Note: It may help to get a heart rate monitor.

#2: Maintain a healthy weight. Being overweight is one of the top risk factors for every disease of the circulatory system. There are a myriad of both direct and indirect ways that obesity negatively impacts your circulatory system, but the bottom line is that the extra fat stresses your heart and circulation. The great news is that the closer you get to a healthy weight range, the lower your risk factors for cardiac disease. If you fill your diet with all the healthy foods mentioned in this chapter and cut back on the unhealthy ones, you're taking a giant leap toward achieving this goal.

#3: Stay hydrated. Say "yes" to water for your heart. Water is the best source of hydration; it regulates blood circulation, helping with digestion and transporting nutrients and oxygen to your cells. If you're not properly hydrated, you can experience irregular heartbeats and you're more likely to have plaque build up in your arteries over time.

#4: Avoid smoking. The toxins your body encounters from smoking can increase your heart rate and blood pressure and decrease your cardiac output over time. Plus, smoking increases your risk of developing blood clots.

#5: Supplements. You'll find a list of specific supplements divided into two groups: one for people who have been diagnosed with high cholesterol but cannot tolerate statins, and one for people with normal cholesterol levels.

Watch Your Sodium Intake

Too much sodium can increase your blood pressure. It's important to follow the guidelines for the amount of sodium that you should be consuming per day: 2,300 milligrams total. However, you shouldn't have more than 1,500 milligrams per day if you fall into any of these categories:

- Over the age of 51
- African-American
- Diagnosed with hypertension
- Diagnosed with diabetes
- Diagnosed with chronic kidney disease

The most common sources of extra sodium are processed or packaged foods. Become cognizant of the nutritional labels on the foods you're eating to get an idea of how much sodium you're consuming each day. You might be shocked! Take strides toward reducing your overall intake right away.

Before we get to Cycle 1: Restore to improve the current state of your circulatory system, take the quiz below. Then, take it again after you've followed my 17 Day Plan; you'll be amazed by your improvement.

Is Your Circulatory System on Its Way to 100 Happy, Healthy Years?

Answer each question honestly; give yourself the designated points for each answer. Add up your total and score yourself.

1. **Are you overweight by 15 pounds or more, based on the charts in Chapter 2?**

    A. Yes ☐ 0 points   B. No ☐ 4 points

2. **Do you get headaches or feel bloated, confused, sluggish, or sleepy after eating?**

    A. Yes ☐ 0 points   B. No ☐ 4 points

3. **Do you have a significant amount of stress in your life?**

    A. Yes ☐ 0 points   B. No ☐ 4 points

4. **Have you ever had a blood clot, a stroke, or a heart attack?**

    A. Yes ☐ 0 points   B. No ☐ 4 points

5. **Do you currently smoke?**

    A. Yes ☐ 0 points   B. No ☐ 4 points

6. **How often do you exercise?**

    A. I don't exercise. ☐ 0 points
    B. I don't exercise, except for light activity like housework. ☐ 1 point

C. I exercise once or twice a week for 30 minutes or longer. ☐ 2 points

D. I exercise three times a week for 30 minutes or longer. ☐ 3 points

E. I exercise more than three times a week for 30 minutes or longer.
☐ 4 points

7. **How often do you experience shortness of breath going up the stairs, flushed cheeks, or headaches?**

A. Frequently, almost daily ☐ 0 points

B. Occasionally, a few times a week ☐ 1 point

C. Seldom, a few times a month ☐ 2 points

D. Rarely ☐ 3 points

E. Never ☐ 4 points

8. **Look over the list of anti-inflammatory foods. How often do you eat those foods?**

A. Never ☐ 0 points

B. I eat one or two servings of those foods weekly. ☐ 1 point

C. I eat four servings of those foods weekly. ☐ 2 points

D. I eat five to six servings of those foods weekly. ☐ 3 points

E. I eat three or more servings of those foods daily. ☐ 4 points

9. **The last time I had my LDL cholesterol tested, it was:**

A. 190 mg/dL and above ☐ 0 points

B. 160 to 189 mg/dL ☐ 1 point

C. 130 to 159 mg/dL ☐ 2 points

D. 100 to 129 mg/dL ☐ 3 points

E. Less than 100 mg/dL ☐ 4 points

10. **The last time I had my HDL cholesterol tested, it was:**

A. lower than 40 mg/dL ☐ 0 points

B. 40 mg/dL and above ☐ 4 points

11. **The last time I had my triglycerides tested, they were:**

A. 500 mg/dL and above ☐ 0 points

B. 200–499 mg/dL ☐ 1 point

C. 150–199 mg/dL ☐ 2 points

D. Less than 150 mg/dL ☐ 4 points

12. **My blood pressure is:**

> A. 160 or higher (upper number) and 100 or higher (lower number)
>   □ 0 points
> B. 140–159 (upper number) and 90–99 (lower number) □ 1 point
> C. 139 or less (upper number) and 89 or less (lower number) □ 4 points

13 **My C-reactive protein (CRP) levels are:**

> A. I don't know □ 0 points
> B. higher than 3.0/L □ 0 points
> C. 1.0 to 2.9/L □ 2 points
> D. lower than 1.0/L □ 4 points

14. **My resting heart rate is: (You can easily check your pulse on the inside of your wrist, below your thumb, or in the carotid artery. This is located in your neck, on either side of your windpipe. But don't push too hard.)**

> A. higher than 100 □ 0 points
> B. 60 to 100 □ 3 points
> C. 40 to 60 □ 4 points

Scoring:

0–12: URGENT; see your doctor ASAP regarding the health of your circulatory system.

13–24: DANGEROUS; change your behavior that's endangering your heart right away.

25–36: MODERATELY RISKY; change your bad heart habits and incorporate more of my techniques that can help improve your heart health.

37–48: AVERAGE; you have room for additional change.

49 AND HIGHER: EXCELLENT; stay on this positive course.

The bottom line: Your heart is your constant companion. It supports you every second of every day. It is, in fact, your life support. I know it's easy to take your ticker for granted. After all, it's a muscle you've never have to purposely flex. But if you neglect it, ignore it, or abuse it, your heart and circulatory system will start to decline and suddenly you'll wish you had paid it some gratitude for its hard work over all those years. So nurture your heart just a little, and it will help you pave the way to your 100th birthday.

CHAPTER 4

Breathe Easy

Watch your kids sometime as they dash up and down stairs or dart across the playing field effortlessly. They don't even need to stop to catch their breath! We grownups, on the other hand, might have to pause mid-activity as we gasp for air. By the time we hit our 40s, breathlessness rears its ugly head more frequently after racing upstairs, running to the gate to catch a flight, or—let's be honest—having sex. If you think it's age catching up with you, think again.

Aging doesn't cause breathlessness. If it did, I wouldn't be able to explain the 80-something-year-old guys I see working out at the gym who are kicking the butts of people 20-plus years younger than they are! Yes, those guys are out there, and they're not gasping for air. You know what often causes breathlessness? The lack of conditioning and good health habits, that's what. If you're someone who walks, jogs, swims, or bikes regularly—and you do not smoke—you have enough respiratory capacity to breathe easy throughout your life. Keep it up! For the rest of you who think you may need a little (or a lot of!) improvement in this area, keep reading.

Respiratory System 101

Each and every day, we breathe in and out about 20,000 times. All this breathing uses every aspect of the respiratory system: the nose, throat, voice box, windpipe, and lungs.

Your lungs resemble upside-down trees. They have branches that lead into air sacs, or alveoli, which deliver oxygen to the blood and remove carbon dioxide.

If the air you breathe is dirty or polluted, the pollutants are expelled, destroyed by digestive juices, or gobbled up by macrophages, a type of immune cell that patrols the body looking for germs to destroy. These actions are examples of the wonderful ways that your respiratory system filters out toxins and self-protects your health.

Yet, there are so many factors that can affect our lung power, both within our bodies and in our environment. Take a bout of flu or pneumonia, for example. In your later years, these infections can put some of your lung capacity out of commission. And if lung power diminishes, you might suffer a heart attack or stroke, since too little oxygen is making its way to your heart or brain. Even eating lots of sugar, thereby aggravating blood sugar levels, hurts your lungs. Excess glucose in the blood creates advanced glycation end-products, those nasty AGEs I mentioned earlier. AGEs cause lung tissue to stiffen and become inflexible, making it harder to breathe.

The lungs are very vulnerable to the outdoor environment, too. Overexposure to environmental gases—I'm talking about cigarette smoke and air pollution—may zap your lung power and accelerate aging. Potential assaults to lung health are all around us, and within us, but fortunately we can guard ourselves from them with some simple but key defenses.

Most Common Lung Problems

Before I get into all the respiratory problems that can develop with age, here are common problems experienced by people of all ages. I mention these because they are often lifestyle related—which means they can be easily avoided.

Asthma. More than 20 million Americans suffer from asthma. It is a long-term, inflammatory lung disease that causes airways to tighten and narrow when an afflicted person comes into contact with irritants such as cigarette smoke, dust, or pet dander.

COPD (chronic obstructive pulmonary disease). This is a common lung disease that makes it very difficult to breathe. Studies have found a major cause of COPD is smoking of any kind, as well as consistent exposure to secondhand smoke. Symptoms include coughing, wheezing, fatigue, and shortness of breath.

Emphysema. This is actually a type of COPD, and smoking is the number-one cause as well. It is what happens when the alveoli (the tiny air sacs throughout your lungs) are damaged, and ultimately destroyed. Patients sometimes won't experience any symptoms at first, but it will often lead to chronic shortness of breath and rapid heartbeat. There are treatment options, but there is no cure.

Bronchitis. Bronchitis is a respiratory disease, and there are actually two types: acute (of shorter duration) and chronic (lasting much longer). It causes a lot of mucus and inflammation to form in the bronchial tubes, which leads the patient to cough up phlegm. Bronchitis is a condition that represents inflammation of the bronchioles, or airways, and is typically caused by viruses and/or bacteria.

Common cold. Colds, which I see in my office on a daily basis, are caused by more than 200 different viruses, which inflame the upper respiratory tract. Common indicators that you have a cold include coughing, sneezing, sore throat, nasal congestion, and headache.

Pneumonia. Pneumonia is an inflammation of the lungs caused by a bacterial or viral infection. Pneumonia causes fever and inflamed lung tissue; it is hard for sufferers to breathe because the lungs have to work harder to transfer oxygen into the bloodstream and remove carbon dioxide from the blood.

How the Lungs and Respiratory System Age

Many factors—including genetics, smoking, pollutants, irritants, and infectious diseases—can cause your lungs and respiratory system to develop problems and age faster than normal. Problems of the respiratory system that involve aging include:

Forced vital capacity (FVC). This refers to the amount of air you can forcibly expel after a big inhalation. This is an important factor: People with healthy lungs have a high FVC. It indicates how well other organs are receiving oxygen, which is required for life. So it's pretty clear: You want to maintain your lung power for good health and longevity.

Interstitial fibrosis. With this condition, fibrous material accumulates in the lungs and thickens the walls of the alveoli. This fibrous material can also obstruct air passages, or bronchioles, to which the air sacs are attached. Symptoms of interstitial fibrosis include shortness of breath, chest pain, and coughing that brings up sputum stained with blood.

With age, other changes occur: Your lung elasticity decreases, stiffness of the chest wall increases, and respiratory muscle strength declines. Cigarette and other types of smoking accelerate all of these age-related declines.

SUPPLEMENTS THAT SUPPORT YOUR RESPIRATORY SYSTEM

B COMPLEX

- **Folic acid:** .4 mg
- **B-12:** 2.4 mcg
- **B-6:** 1.3mg

Why? Vitamin B-12 and folic acid (another type of B vitamin) help your body methylate properly, and balancing your DNA methylation is a huge factor in preventing and delaying aging of your lungs and respiratory system. I recommend you take a B-complex vitamin in conjunction with eating plenty of foods rich in these vitamins.

All of this sounds a little depressing, right? It doesn't have to be. As I mentioned earlier, in many ways, the respiratory system can grow healthier and stronger with age. Your lungs are highly sensitive to methylation, a process that, when balanced, occurs within the DNA of cells and prevents abnormalities in how DNA functions. When unbalanced, DNA methylation is serious business and can lead to cancer, including lung cancer. To prevent serious lung diseases, we've got to make sure our bodies are methylating properly. You can do this easily by making sure you take in adequate supplies of vitamin B-12 and folic acid. Both nutrients are key in ensuring balance in your cells' methylation. Folic acid, in particular, is vital for cellular growth and regeneration. This vitamin is abundant in the following foods:

Foods High in Folic Acid

Dark leafy greens (collard greens, kale, mustard greens, spinach, Romaine lettuce, turnip greens)

Asparagus

Broccoli

Citrus fruits

Beans and lentils

Avocado

Okra

Brussels sprouts

Seeds and nuts

Cauliflower

Beets

Corn

Celery

Carrots

Squash

Vitamin B-12 is involved in the metabolism of every cell of the human body, especially affecting DNA synthesis and regulation. You need only a small amount—about two micrograms—of B-12 per day, but you must have it. A short supply of B-12 can lead to anemia, nerve damage, and cognitive problems. Left untreated, a severe deficiency can cause increasingly abnormal blood cell division, potentially even leading to cancer.

As you get older, it's tougher for the body to absorb vitamin B-12, due in part to a reduction in the amount of stomach acid we produce. Medical experts estimate that up to 30 percent of people age 50 and over are affected by this stomach acid decline and subsequent lessening in ability to absorb B-12 and other vitamins. After the age of 60, one in 10 people in North America are thought to be deficient in vitamin B-12. You can counteract this deficiency by supplementing with a B-complex vitamin. You can also obtain this vitamin from the following foods:

Foods High in Vitamin B-12

Clams

Oysters

Mussels

Fish

Lobster
Crab
Beef
Lamb
Cheese
Eggs
Yogurt
Cereals and plant-based foods fortified with vitamin B-12

Supportive Strategies

The Anti-Aging Essentials and
Your Respiratory System

#1: Movement. Right now I'm going to talk specifically about the simple act of walking, but not just any little stroll down the street. How fast—or how slowly—you normally walk may predict how long you'll live, according to a study published in the *Journal of the American Medical Association*. In this particular study, researchers clocked the walking speed of more than 34,000 people, age 65 years and older.

The subjects who averaged 2.25 miles per hour or faster lived longer than those who walked more slowly. Now, I'm not necessarily saying this means that if you increase your walking speed you'll automatically live longer. More importantly, if you notice you simply can't speed up, that could be an indicator that you have an underlying health issue. Try picking up your walking speed during Cycle 1 and if you find yourself really struggling, have a talk with your doctor about what may be going on.

#2: Maintain a healthy weight. Excess weight puts more stress on your lungs and compromises all respiratory muscles, making them work harder and less efficiently. Here's where I direct you back to my 17 Day Diet for help. It is a four-cycle program designed to take weight off rapidly. The diet is nutritionally sound, is easy to follow, and it works. But whatever nutrition and exercise program you choose, take it seriously and lose the extra pounds.

#3: *Stay hydrated.* Drinking plenty of water every day helps maintain a healthy, thin consistency to the mucus lining your airways and lungs. Dehydration can cause that mucus to thicken and get sticky, which slows down overall respiration and makes you more susceptible to illness.

#4: *Avoid smoking.* Smoking damages lung and respiratory health by inducing inflammation, speeding oxidative stress in respiratory cells, and even causing cell death, potentially taking you down the road toward emphysema, chronic lung disease (which in turn increases the risk of pneumonia and heart failure), chronic bronchitis, and lung cancer.

There are numerous methods to quit smoking, and I included several resources in the Appendix of this book. The trick is to keep trying until you find one that works for you. Brad, a patient of mine, was a three-pack-a-day smoker who wanted to quit after his first grandchild was born. He had been smoking for nearly 30 years at the time.

When the urge to smoke struck, he would get up and take a walk around the block. He tried nicotine gum, but it gave him headaches. He made a flavored substitute by drenching toothpicks in cinnamon oil and sucking on them instead of smoking. To stay motivated, he kept his family in his thoughts as much as possible. All of this took a few tries, but ultimately Brad was successful, and he hasn't had any respiratory problems in three years.

If you've tried to quit before, it's time to try again, because the single best thing you can do for your lungs is to stop smoking. Smoking does great damage to your respiratory system, but the good news is that this damage can be undone.

Remember: Even if you've *never* picked up a cigarette, cigar, or pipe, you may still be breathing in an alarming amount of pollutants every day. So, strengthening your respiratory system is helpful even for nonsmokers because you'll be armed against all possible invaders: allergens, bacteria, and viruses. Plus, you don't want to be tethered to an oxygen machine when you're 100 years old, do you? Strong lungs are a key component to overall good health as we age.

#5: *Supplements.* Make sure your multivitamin has the recommended amounts of B vitamins I mention above. If not, you should add an extra B-complex supplement to your regimen.

Learn yoga breathing techniques. Are you a shallow breather? You might be if most of your breaths come from your chest area. I suggest learning to take deep, long breaths, sending fresh oxygen deep into the bottom of your lungs. This not only helps your lungs function better, but it can also bring on a sense of calm. You'll find descriptions of a yoga deep breathing technique called *Breath of Fire* in the Appendix, and it's included in your Restore 17 Day Plan. You'll also see a *Diaphragmatic Breathing Technique* in the Appendix, which teaches you how to breathe into your belly, thus flexing and strengthening your diaphragm. This can be quite renewing, and is excellent exercise for your lungs. Over time, it can help increase your lung capacity.

Stretch your chest. I encourage you to expand and stretch the muscles in your chest, which can also help you send more oxygen deeper into your lungs. The Appendix offers explanations of a *Standing Chest Expansion* and *Cobra Stretches*, both of which accomplish this.

Challenge your lungs. Simple yet challenging exercises like breathing through a straw can improve your lung function by increasing your lung capacity. Other activities that challenge your lungs in a good way are singing, playing wind instruments, and swimming. Overall, I want you to become more aware of your breathing so you can improve it over time and have strong lungs for a lifetime.

Breathe steam. Especially if you suffer from chronic bronchitis, you should breathe steam on a regular basis to loosen up the thick mucus your lungs naturally produce when they're trying to rid themselves of infection. The goal is to get the mucus back to a thin, healthy consistency. When I breathe steam, I like to include a few drops of essential oil like eucalyptus, not only for the pleasing scent, but because they may help purify the lungs. Just taking a steamy shower can achieve this goal.

Consider chiropractic care. After having a chiropractic adjustment, many people comment along the lines of, "I feel like I'm taking in more air." One study on over 5,000 people showed that chiropractic intervention improved overall breathing in 25 percent of the study participants. If you choose this route, discuss it with your general doctor and work with him or her to find a chiropractor and coordinate treatment. I don't recommend seeking chiropractic treatments without first alerting your physician.

Before you begin the Cycle 1: Restore 17 Day Plan, take this quiz. Then, retake it after you've completed the 17 days. Your improvements might just surprise you!

Is Your Respiratory System on Its Way to 100 Happy, Healthy Years?

Answer the following questions and give yourself the points associated with your response. Add up your total score to see how you did.

---

1. **Have you been having shortness of breath or breathlessness?**

    A. Yes ☐ 0 points   B. No ☐ 4 points

---

2. **Do you get shortness of breath with:**

    A. rest ☐ 0 points
    B. minimal activities ☐ 1 point
    C. moderate activities ☐ 2 points
    D. strenuous activities ☐ 3 points
    E. I do not experience shortness of breath. ☐ 4 points

---

3. **Do you have a chronic cough?**

    A. Yes ☐ 0 points   B. No ☐ 4 points

---

4. **How often do you eat foods high in B-12 (such as eggs, cheese, seafood, and yogurt)?**

    A. Never ☐ 0 points
    B. Once or twice per week ☐ 1 point
    C. Three or four times per week ☐ 3 points
    D. Every day ☐ 4 points

---

5. **Have you recently coughed up blood?**

    A. Yes ☐ 0 points   B. No ☐ 4 points

---

6. **Do you ever experience wheezing when you exert yourself (such as when you exercise or go up stairs)?**

    A. Yes ☐ 0 points   B. No ☐ 4 points

7. **How often do you eat colorful fruits and vegetables?**

    A. Never □ 0 points
    B. Once per week, on average □ 1 point
    C. A couple of times per week, on average □ 2 points
    D. Daily □ 4 points

8. **How many days of work have you missed in the past year due to lung problems?**

    A. A month or longer □ 0 points
    B. Three weeks □ 1 point
    C. Two weeks □ 2 points
    D. None □ 4 points

9. **Do you currently smoke cigarettes, cigars, or a pipe?**

    A. Yes □ 0 points   B. No □ 4 points

10. **If you are not a current smoker, do you have a history of 10 years or more of smoking one or more packs a day?**

    A. Yes □ 0 points   B. No □ 4 points

11. **How often are you exposed to secondhand smoke?**

    A. Frequently □ 0 points
    B. Occasionally □ 1 point
    C. Never □ 4 points

12. **How often are you exposed to pollutants or toxins, such as air pollution, dust, or fumes?**

    A. Frequently □ 0 points
    B. Occasionally □ 1 point
    C. Never □ 4 points

13. **Have you ever been exposed to asbestos?**

    A. Yes □ 0 points   B. No □ 4 points

14. **Do you get many colds, and do your colds usually last longer than a week?**

    A. Yes □ 0 points   B. No □ 4 points

0–11: URGENT; see your doctor ASAP about the health of your respiratory system.

12–22: DANGEROUS; stop the behavior that's hurting your lungs immediately.

23–33: MODERATELY RISKY; start incorporating more of my recommendations that can improve your lungs.

34–44: AVERAGE; you have room for additional change.

45–56: EXCELLENT; stay on this positive course.

Dr. Mike's Thyme Tea Recipe

Thyme is an inexpensive herb that was used in ancient times by the Egyptians, Greeks, and Romans for medicinal and ritualistic purposes. Make a cup of thyme tea part of your daily ritual for strong respiration, thanks to its thymol, a potent antioxidant. Added bonus: It's been shown to soothe coughs and bronchitis!

2 cups water
2 tablespoons fresh thyme OR 1 tablespoon dried thyme

Bring the water just to a boil on the stove or in the microwave.

Finely chop the thyme, put inside a tea ball,* and add to a cup.

Pour hot water over the herbs, and let steep for at least five minutes.

*If you don't have a tea ball, strain out the leaves after they have steeped.

Enjoy!

Yield: 2 cups

I truly don't want you to be on oxygen when you are much older; being tethered to a tank is no way to go about life, and our goal here is to help you feel fit and active when you're 100 years old! By taking these simple steps earlier in life, you are setting yourself up for many years of healthier, heartier lungs. So to keep your respiratory system strong, don't smoke, avoid exposure to pollutants, stay active, and eat healthful foods—all easy-to-follow lifestyle measures you can take to ensure a healthy, vibrant respiratory system.

CHAPTER 5

Brainpower

When I "grow up," I want to be as mentally alert as my patient Rhonda. In her 80s, she still has an excitement about life and the enriching discoveries she makes daily.

I asked her one day, "How do you keep so mentally fit?" Rhonda has had many hobbies over the years. She's active with friends and with her church. She's always trying new things, from foods to television programs. She even takes different routes on errands to ensure she never lives life on autopilot.

People like Rhonda seem to defy aging. She exudes gusto and youth. She's physically healthy, has laser-sharp faculties, is almost always radiant, and her life is filled with great friends and family members on whom she can rely. Don't you just want to bottle whatever it is she has?

Well, it doesn't exactly come in a bottle, but it's all yours if you just put in a little effort. In this chapter, I'll tell you how to focus those efforts. When you take care of your brain and nervous system, feelings of happiness, hope, optimism, and youthfulness will naturally follow. If you make the simple changes I suggest, I'm willing to bet you'll see and feel some pretty amazing improvements over the course of just 17 days.

Nervous System 101

Atop the spinal cord, not unlike a flower upon its stem, sits the most complex and amazing object on Earth: the human brain. This moist, pinkish-gray organ is the human control center because it regulates everything we do: thought, reason, intuition, emotion, sight, hearing, touch, movement, speech, memory, creativity—everything, in fact, that makes us human. The brain is the most vital organ in the body. So you've got to protect it!

Envision your brain as your body's mission command center. Now, your nervous system is similar to a communications system, taking messages back and forth from the brain to every other part of your body. And your spinal cord is the superhighway, acting as a route for these communications, with its tiny nerves that branch out to every organ and system in your body.

For example, say you step out in front of a moving car. The nerves in your skin shoot a message of "jump back" to your brain. The brain then sends a message telling the muscles in your legs to get on that curb and out of harm's way. Luckily, this neurological relay race takes place instantaneously, in much less time than it takes for me to explain it.

There are three interconnecting parts of the nervous system:

The central nervous system (CNS). This consists of the brain and spinal cord. Overall, the CNS dispatches nerve impulses and analyzes information from your sense organs (ears, eyes, and so forth). When the CNS is working at top-notch efficiency, you can hear clearly, see optimally, smell the most minute odors and scents, and be very sensitive to touch.

The peripheral nervous system (PNS). Imagine this system as tree-like branches of nerves spreading out from your spinal cord to every part of your body. The PNS is assigned to carry nerve impulses from the CNS to your muscles and glands. Disease, physical injury, poor nutrition, and exposure to toxins or poisons can cause nerve damage in the PNS, sometimes resulting in a person losing feeling or even becoming paralyzed.

The autonomic nervous system (ANS). This system controls breathing, heartbeat, digestion, blood pressure, and other bodily functions that occur automatically, or without us thinking about them. The ANS is divided into two different parts: the sympathetic and parasympathetic systems.

The parasympathetic system sends signals to the body to slow down and work at a normal pace (rest and digest), whereas the sympathetic system helps accelerate the body when you need to be active or you're under stress (as when you might need to flee from an assailant, as in the term "fight or flight"). A good example is blood pressure; if it rises suddenly, sympathetic activity increases and parasympathetic activity decreases. By producing opposite effects, the two systems keep the body in equilibrium.

When the ANS goes on the fritz for some reason, it may cause serious, often debilitating problems, such as abnormal blood pressure, heart trouble, difficulty breathing and swallowing, and erectile dysfunction in men. Obviously, keeping this system in peak condition prevents many health complications.

How the Nervous System Ages

When I was in med school, we were taught that the central nervous system couldn't repair itself following damage due to trauma such as head injury or disorders such as Alzheimer's disease, nor could the brain regenerate new brain cells. Essentially, we learned that the brain gradually degenerates over a lifetime. Fortunately, that thinking has been turned upside down. Now we know the brain and central nervous systems have the ability to regenerate. This is fantastic news, because it means you're not destined to suffer with brain and nervous system problems like memory lapses, loss of judgment, lack of clarity, or even dementia.

But, yes, many facets of the nervous system can undergo changes as we age, so let's talk about those for a moment. First, the nerve cells in your brain and spinal cord tend to shrink, so they don't transmit messages as rapidly. As nerve cells degenerate, waste products can accumulate in the brain, causing plaque, which increases your risk of stroke, Alzheimer's, and other serious issues.

When nerves aren't working up to par, your senses are affected. Take hearing, for example. It's not just all that hair in your grandpa's ears that make it difficult for him to hear! As you age, the inner workings of your ear tend to weaken, and your hearing will likely decline. I encourage my patients to get annual hearing tests so they can keep track of this decline and decide on a treatment option, such as hearing aids, if necessary.

This process can start to affect your balance, too, since your equilibrium has lots to do with your inner ear. Our fancy name for this age-related hearing loss is presbycusis. Another fancy name to keep in mind, since it's also common as we get up in years, is tinnitus. It's a nonstop, abnormal (often high-pitched) ear noise. If you have symptoms, talk to your doctor about the best solution for you.

Aging also affects vision. Almost every one of my patients over the age of 55 needs glasses at least sometimes. That can mean just a simple pair of reading glasses, or it can mean bifocals.

Most commonly, people find it harder to focus on objects or text up close, a condition called presbyopia. Some people can't tolerate glare as well, and others may even have more trouble seeing when it's very dark or very bright. It's no fun and sometimes embarrassing not being able to read a menu, but the solution could be as simple as a pair of reading glasses, so keep up those annual eye doctor appointments to make sure you're in the know about how your eyesight is doing.

As nerves break down, your taste is affected, too. I know it's a little sad to think about not being able to taste your favorite foods (or wines), but part of getting older is losing some of your taste buds. Between the ages of 40 and 60, the number of taste buds in our mouth decreases. Plus, the ones left behind actually shrink in size, so you do lose some of your ability to taste, specifically salty and sweet foods.

Additionally, less saliva is produced as you get older. This can cause dry mouth, and can make swallowing more difficult. Saliva is important to digestion, so with less saliva, digestion is less efficient.

Aging also impacts your sense of smell. The gradual loss of smell typically happens after the age of 70. It may be caused by the process of losing nerve endings inside the nose or by certain medications. As they get older, many people take more medication, some of which can impair smell, such as estrogen, nasal decongestants (with long-term use), and zinc supplements. There's no real "cure" for the loss of smell due to aging. Prevention, while you can still sniff optimally, is your best bet.

Then there's memory. It's the one thing no one wants to lose, ever. Even young people forget things here and there. I mean, who hasn't forgotten a password to access computer information? A personal identification number at the ATM? Where they parked their car or left their keys? As you age, your memory gets even worse, especially if you haven't taken care of your brain and nervous system in a long time. One reason is that the brain naturally shrinks, losing up to 10 percent of its weight by age 90. This is caused by the shrinkage of nerve cells in the brain and is considered a normal consequence of aging. But with significant shrinkage, there can be dementia, seizures, and a condition called aphasia, in which a person can't talk or is unable to understand language.

By now, I know you're thinking "eek, old age isn't fun!" But hold on. There's plenty you can do now to prevent—or at least slow down—all this.

BRAIN ATTACK!

The risk of having a stroke, or what you can think of as a "brain attack," definitely increases as you get older. There are two types of stroke, ischemic (when a blood clot stops blood from being able to make its way to the brain, thus shutting off your oxygen supply to that section of the brain) and hemorrhagic (when a blood vessel in your brain actually bursts). They're both extremely serious medical emergencies and can lead to permanent brain damage. You can significantly reduce your risk for stroke, even if you have family members that have suffered strokes, by keeping your cholesterol low, your weight in a healthy range, not smoking, and preventing diabetes.

SUPPLEMENTS THAT SUPPORT YOUR NERVOUS SYSTEM

- **Vitamin C:** 1,000 mg daily
- **Vitamin E:** 200 IUs daily
- **Fish oil:** 3 grams daily
- **B Complex:**

    Folic Acid: .4 mg
    B-12: 2.4 mcg
    B-6: 1.3mg
- **Selenium:** .2 mg
- **Turmeric:** 750 mg daily

Why: A 2004 Johns Hopkins study of more than 4,700 elderly participants found a reduced incidence of Alzheimer's disease in those given a combination of vitamin C and vitamin E supplements. In addition, DHA (found in fish oil) has been shown to boost brainpower. So especially if you aren't eating foods high in DHA, you should supplement with fish oil.

Turmeric is an Indian spice with many medicinal purposes. In a study from the University of California, Los Angeles, curcumin, a potent antioxidant and anti-inflammatory compound found in turmeric, helped reduce the accumulation of amyloid protein plaques in mice, the same plaques seen in Alzheimer's disease patients. Previous research has shown a low incidence of Alzheimer's among elders in India, possibly due to turmeric's popularity in Indian cuisine. It just so happens that, in my opinion, turmeric also tastes delicious. I recommend using it in chicken, fish, or veggie dishes for a light, curry-like flavor. However, if you don't like it or don't think you'll use it often, you can take it in pill form.

B vitamins work together as a group to support the nervous system. For example, folic acid lowers homocysteine only in the presence of adequate levels of vitamins B-6 and B-12. Low levels of B-12 and B-6, as well as low levels of folic acid, have been linked to Alzheimer's disease and cognitive decline.

Another brain-healthy antioxidant is selenium. French researchers found that it may halt some of the mental decline that occurs with age; a long-term study revealed that as blood levels of selenium drop over time in older people, mental function suffers as well. This study involved nearly 1,400 people who were followed up with after two years, and again after nine years. It was at the nine-year follow-up that the connection between selenium and cognitive decline was discovered. The researchers believe that selenium may prevent oxidative stress to the brain, which may be responsible for some of the mental decline that comes with aging.

THE CONNECTION BETWEEN DENTAL AND MENTAL . . .

A recent study showed that folks who don't take great care of their teeth and gums are more likely to have cognitive problems, such as difficulties with memory. Researchers worked with more than 2,000 men and women over the age of 60, all with periodontitis (gum disease). They tested their memories and found that the higher the level of bacteria causing their gum disease, the worse they did on the memory tests. And the less bacteria they had, the better they performed on the cognitive tests.

So follow your dentist's advice by flossing daily and brush your teeth for a full two minutes at least once a day. Not that pretty teeth weren't enough of a motivation—but now you can think about preserving your brain health every time you brush and floss!

Number-One Strategy: Fight Free Radicals

Weighing in at just three pounds, the brain accounts for only 2 percent of your body's total weight, yet it uses up to *half* of the body's total oxygen. It takes a lot of O_2 to keep those wheels turning up there! With this high metabolic activity, the brain is susceptible to damage from free radicals, the destructive by-products of normal body processes, and is thus very vulnerable to oxidative stress, as well as to inflammation. Over time, all of this damage to the brain can affect cognitive function, memory, mood, movement, and your overall quality of life.

The easiest way to keep your brain and entire CNS (if you've already forgotten that CNS stands for "central nervous system," read on so you can get your brain operating optimally!) from aging is to increase anti-oxidants in your diet through such foods as colorful fruits (grapes, apples, cantaloupe, and berries) and green leafy vegetables, five servings a day. This may sound familiar, since I just advised you in the circulatory system chapter to eat these fruits and vegetables; these foods really help you across the board, and the good news is that when you're eating them to help one system you're giving a boost to all of the others!

People who don't eat a lot of the B-complex vitamin, folic acid, found primarily in leafy green vegetables (yes, I'm talking to you, delinquent veggie eaters), tend to have elevated levels of homocysteine, which has been linked to cognitive decline. Studies of older individuals found that elevated homocysteine levels with folic acid deficiencies were associated with cognitive impairment. That's no good! But how amazing that it's within your control to change. I'd like to see you getting most of your folic acid from food, but I suggest you also take a B-complex vitamin as backup.

I'm not giving you permission to become a lush, but my next suggestion is that you enjoy a glass of wine on a regular basis. Red wine has resveratrol, a powerful antioxidant found in grape skin. Studies have shown that resveratrol protects cells by mopping up free radicals, while others show it actually encourages nerve cells to regrow. It also turns off a gene that activates inflammation. So, cheers (within reason)! One of my hobbies outside of work is collecting and drinking fine red wine, so I attend wine tastings with friends when I can. How great that I found a hobby that also helps my nervous system—win/win!

The Anti-Aging Essentials and Your Nervous System

#1: Movement. You'll see in the "Use it or lose it" section the amazing ways exercise can anti-age your brain, boost creativity, and make you think more clearly right now!

#2: Maintain a healthy weight. Studies have revealed a relationship between brain volume, or size, and BMI, body mass index. Study participants whose BMI fell in the overweight or obese category were found to have smaller brains overall. Furthermore, research indicates that being overweight puts you at a higher risk of getting Alzheimer's later in life.

#3: Stay hydrated. Water your brain for better memory! No, don't pour it on your head. Drink it! Did you know that even a little dehydration can blur your thinking? I've had so many patients fear they were surely losing their minds but really, they were just dehydrated. Get enough water—at least six to eight glasses of pure water daily—so that your urine looks pale at all times. Sip, don't chug. Your body can't absorb more than one cup in 20 minutes.

If you don't like plain drinking water, do something—whatever it takes—to make it more palatable to you, such as adding a squeeze of lemon, some sliced cucumbers or strawberries . . . or have sparkling water instead.

#4: Avoid smoking. Researchers recently discovered that one of the chemicals in tobacco products actually causes immune cells within the brain to attack healthy brain tissue, causing damage. That's right—this inflammatory immune response can cause brain damage.

#5: Supplements. Check out the section of this chapter that features my list of supplements that specifically support your brain and nervous system over time.

AN APPLE A DAY KEEPS A STROKE AWAY?

An apple a day does keep doctors (like me) away, but could it also help prevent you from having a stroke? It's true: Apples and other fruits and vegetables with white flesh (pears, bananas, and cauliflower are some examples) appear to decrease the risk of stroke, according to a study from the Netherlands that was published in 2011. Apples also provide catechins and quercetin, potent natural substances called flavonoids that might help prevent various types of cancer. Whether you're into Granny Smith or Red Delicious, crunch on an apple every day to help protect your brain.

Along with antioxidants, make sure you're supplementing with omega-3 fatty acids with DHA. This supplement may be beneficial in easing bad moods, rejuvenating the brain, enhancing memory, protecting against the development of Alzheimer's and it may even have a positive effect on vision. The recommended dosage for omega-3 fatty acids is 300 to 500 milligrams and 800 to 1,100 milligrams of DHA daily. Plus, consider including foods high in polyunsaturated fats (known as PUFAs) in your everyday diet.

Foods High in Polyunsaturated Fats

Nuts and seeds

Walnuts
Sunflower seeds
Flaxseed
Sesame seeds
Fatty fish
Salmon
Mackerel
Herring
Trout
Vegetable oils
Safflower oil

Supportive Strategies:
Use It or Lose It

Aside from filling your diet with antioxidants, there are other ways you can revitalize and rejuvenate your nervous system. I'll sum this up for you in four words: Use it or lose it.

Think of physical exercise (cardio, weight training, and any other physical activity) and mental exercise (doing crossword puzzles, problem-solving, and intellectual pursuits) as the dynamic duo in brain health. When it comes to physical exercise, what's good for the body is good for the brain—and that includes working out on a regular basis. Exercise pumps more oxygenated blood to your brain. That helps you think more clearly and creatively.

Ever been to an aerobics dance class? If you have, good, because this type of workout involves complicated motor skills. That means your brain is working on a mental level to learn the skills, while your body is boosting oxygen to the brain. The net effect is that your brain builds stronger connections and thus is able to process more information.

EXERCISE YOUR WAY TO STRAIGHT A'S?

We know that regular exercise keeps the mind sharp in older adults, but a recent study demonstrates the same benefits in young adults. College students who met the Centers for Disease Control and Prevention's activity requirements—leisurely physical activity at least five times per week for 30 minutes or vigorous physical activity for 20 minutes at least three times per week— were found to have better working memory capacity than students who did not meet the requirements. Whether you're still in school or not, you're taking in new information every day; why not improve your ability to remember all that info simply by moving your body?

Physical exercise also improves reaction time, meaning how long it takes you to react to an unexpected situation, such as grabbing your toddler before she steps into the street.

Work out and your brain will make more neurotransmitters—brain chemicals that affect mood, memory, and the transmission of messages throughout your body. Diseases such as Parkinson's are caused by a short supply of neurotransmitters in the nervous system. Exercise may have an important protective effect against such conditions.

Staying active protects your aging brain in many other ways, primarily by producing "growth factors"—proteins that help give birth to new brain cells. These growth factors create stronger connections among brain cells, which means that information, problem-solving, and other mental functions are transacted lickety-split.

As for mental activities, there's plenty you can do to keep your brain youthful. Go Internet surfing, for example. When you surf the Internet, you activate key centers in your brain that control decision-making and reasoning. Those few clicks may be more mentally engaging than reading, say UCLA scientists—but only in folks with prior Internet-surfing experience. MRI results showed almost three times more brain activity in regular Internet searchers than in newbies. In other words, the more you go "surfing," the more cognitive power you can build over time.

So, fire up the computer, log on, and search to the end of the Internet (or as far as you can get in 20 minutes) for any subject that intrigues you. You could see what your favorite actress wore to the Oscars, plan your next vacation, or learn something about your health. No matter what you search for, your brain can benefit from your surfing!

As for other mental activities, you could knock 10 years off your brain age by doing a crossword puzzle, playing Scrabble, or playing other "brain games." Maybe your latest cell phone game addiction is actually a good thing! Researchers created one experiment in which 3,000 older adults performed cognitively challenging activities, such as crossword puzzles. They did the activities 10 times, for an hour or more each time. Want to venture a guess at how much they were able to improve their brain functioning? Did they turn back the clock by two years? Five years? Believe it or not, by the end of the study, these participants' brains were functioning at the level of someone 10 years younger. So, what are you waiting for? Grab yourself a Sudoku puzzle, word puzzle, or similar activity and put that brain to work!

Try some brain aerobics, too. Remember my patient Rhonda, who would take different routes to do her errands just to keep her brain engaged? She was on to something. By making yourself do things differently, you'll activate new brain circuits and enhance the production of neurotrophins, growth factors in the brain. Here's an example: If you are normally right-handed, switch to writing left-handed for a bit. (You may not want this to be an important document—maybe start with a grocery list!) Suddenly your brain is confronted with an engaging task that's interesting, challenging, and fun (and probably frustrating—but that works to your benefit). Other tips: Take a different route on your way to work. Try a recipe you've never made before instead of the same one your family has been making for decades. Listen to a different music genre. Maneuver from one room to another room in your home with your eyes closed. Rearrange your kitchen cupboards, forcing you to break old habits of always reaching for certain dishes or utensils in one place.

Also, try a mental exercise in relaxation. I'm talking about meditation. It has been shown to have some pretty exciting effects on the brain. Researchers report that those who meditated for about 30 minutes a day for eight weeks improved their memory, bolstered their self-esteem, and reduced stress levels. They even conducted brain scans on the participants to prove that the meditating patients had additional gray matter in the learning and memory center of the brain, as well as less gray matter in the area associated with stress. (More gray matter means higher functioning in that area.) The control group showed no changes. Better memory and less stress? Meditation is a win-win!

DR. MIKE'S MEDITATION

In case you've never meditated before, I'll share some tips from my own experience. Sit with your back erect. Don't try to meditate while lying on your back, because you might go to sleep. While sleep is also relaxing, meditation brings on a peaceful feeling while you are fully alert and conscious. Your sense of awareness should be heightened, which can't happen if you're out cold.

I recommend meditating early in the morning. Some say the ideal time is 3 a.m., but I feel it is more important to get a full night's sleep and then be fully awake, so I meditate at 6:30 a.m. Don't eat before meditating, because a heavy meal could make you lethargic.

One-Pointed Concentration: When you sit down to meditate for the first time, you will probably be painfully aware of how cluttered your mind is. Work toward getting your mind to calm down to the point that you can concentrate on a single thought instead of holding several ideas in your head at the same time. A key way to focus your mind and concentrate on a single thought is through the use of a mantra, the repetition of a sacred word. For example, you might repeat the mantra "ohm" a certain number of times.

Silent Mind: After you've practiced concentration and learned to focus on one thing at a time, you can proceed to the next stage: no thought at all. Achieving a silent mind is difficult, but it's a powerful experience after you master it.

Through meditation, you can attain the power to control your thoughts, and on occasion stop them completely. Don't be discouraged if you can't do it perfectly right away. It takes time and practice, but is a powerful way to boost your brainpower and alleviate stress as well.

The brain may not be a muscle that you can work out at the gym, but as I'm demonstrating, using it over and over broadens the brain connections between neurons. Another way to accomplish this is to learn a foreign language. Research shows that this actually builds your brain. It doesn't have to mean signing up for a time-intensive or expensive class;

just get a foreign-language teaching CD and listen to it in the car during your commute.

Not into language? Well, how about listening to some music? I recommend Mozart, since brain studies show that it excites and enhances firing patterns in the brain that are used to process and execute complex tasks requiring advanced reasoning, such as math and engineering. In other words, it could enhance your intelligence.

Keep your brain alive and those neurons firing by constantly learning. Whether you're studying economics or learning how to sew a skirt, taking classes is great for your brain. Consider enrolling in an adult education class to reenergize your brain and thinking skills. Nowadays you don't even need to leave your home, because there are so many online courses.

THINKING AND YOUR THYROID

People who are low in thyroid hormone (hypothyroidism) can experience memory loss and fuzzy thinking. And guess when thyroid production declines? As we age. Many women experience forgetfulness during menopause for this reason. But there are treatment options, so get a complete thyroid panel to test your levels. The sooner you get it checked, the better!

Before we get to Cycle 1: Restore and the 17 Day Plan to improve the functioning of your nervous system, take the quiz below. Then, take it again after 17 days to measure your improvement.

Is Your Nervous System on Its Way to 100 Happy, Healthy Years?

Answer the following questions and give yourself the points assigned to each question. Tally up your total and see how you scored.

1. **Is your memory noticeably declining?**

    A. Yes, quite a bit ☐ 0 points

    B. Somewhat ☐ 2 points

    C. Not at all ☐ 4 points

2. **Is it difficult for you to remember names and phone numbers?**

   A. Yes, quite a bit ☐ 0 points
   B. Somewhat ☐ 2 points
   C. Not at all ☐ 4 points

3. **Have you lost your enthusiasm for your favorite activities?**

   A. Yes, quite a bit ☐ 0 points
   B. Somewhat ☐ 2 points
   C. Not at all ☐ 4 points

4. **How often do you use turmeric or take a turmeric supplement?**

   A. Never ☐ 0 points
   B. Once in a while ☐ 2 points
   C. Daily ☐ 4 points

5. **Is poor vision affecting your daily life?**

   A. Yes ☐ 0 points   B. No ☐ 4 points

6. **Do you eat a poor diet?**

   A. Definitely; I eat a lot of junk food and fatty foods. ☐ 0 points
   B. I eat some junk food and try to eat more fruits and vegetables.
      ☐ 2 points
   C. I am conscious of my diet and eat mostly natural foods—lots of
      fruits, vegetables, and whole grains. ☐ 4 points

7. **Do you take supplemental antioxidants?**

   A. Never ☐ 0 points
   B. Occasionally ☐ 2 points
   C. Every day ☐ 4 points

8. **How often do you surf the Internet?**

   A. Never ☐ 0 points
   B. Occasionally ☐ 2 points
   C. All the time ☐ 4 points

9. **Is there a history of stroke in your family?**

   A. Yes—parent, sibling, or grandparent ☐ 0 points

   B. Yes, but in more distant relatives such as cousins ☐ 2 points

   C. No, not to my knowledge ☐ 4 points

10. **How often do you meditate?**

    A. Never ☐ 0 points

    B. Occasionally ☐ 2 points

    C. Every day ☐ 4 points

11. **How are your oral hygiene habits, on average?**

    A. I never floss, but brush regularly. ☐ 0 points

    B. I brush twice daily and floss when I remember. ☐ 2 points

    C. I brush two to three times per day and floss once daily. ☐ 4 points

12. **How much water do you drink on a daily basis?**

    A. Almost none ☐ 0 points

    B. Two to three cups ☐ 2 points

    C. Eight cups or more ☐ 4 points

13. **How often do you challenge your mind with quizzes and games?**

    A. Never ☐ 0 points

    B. A few times a week ☐ 2 points

    C. Most days of the week ☐ 4 points

14. **Are you currently taking a class or learning something new, such as a language?**

    A. No ☐ 0 points

    B. Yes ☐ 4 points

Scoring:

0–14: URGENT; if you have recently noticed a sharp decline in your memory or cognitive abilities, speak with your doctor about it. Otherwise, make immediate changes in your habits affecting your nervous system.

15–24: DANGEROUS; you should change your ways ASAP.

25–34: RISKY; start incorporating my suggested techniques that help your brain.

35–44: AVERAGE; you have room for additional change.

45–54: EXCELLENT; stay on this positive course.

Here's the deal: Your brain is a beautiful thing; what an incredible gift! I really wish I could tell you that your nervous system is always going to operate as well as it did when you were 29, but I can't. However, there is so much you can do to tip the odds in your favor that you'll be living 100 happy, healthy years with the same joie de vivre that my patient Rhonda will likely have for many years to come. Push the limits of your brain-power every single day, and you'll surely reap the rewards both now and later in life.

CHAPTER 6

Cycle 1: 17 Day Plan

Restoring your primary systems—circulatory, respiratory, and nervous—to a baseline level of good health is the central goal of Cycle 1: Restore. In the next 17 days, assuming you follow this plan, you'll experience marked improvements in your cardiovascular performance, lung health, and mental acuity. Here are the specific goals to keep in mind as you go.

Goals of Cycle 1: Restore

Bring resting heart rate into healthy range
Improve cholesterol levels
Lower CRP (C-reactive protein) levels
Lose weight
Increase physical strength
Increase lung capacity
Deepen breathing
Prevent lung infections
Improve memory
Prevent dementia
Boost creativity
Enhance the five senses

If you scored low on any of the three Cycle 1: Restore quizzes, make sure you're following the supportive strategies for those particular systems every day, even above and beyond what you'll find in this 17 Day Plan. There are some additional ways for you to see profound change in your health as a result of the work you're doing in the next 17 days. First, you can perform an at-home cholesterol test (readily available online) before you begin and again on day 18. Another option, depending on your doctor and insurance coverage, is to request a CRP (C-reactive protein) test before and after the 17 days. A CRP test is often done in conjunction with a cholesterol test at your doctor's lab . . . so it can be a two-for-one!

You can also measure your current lung capacity by having your doctor perform a simple pulmonary function test or you can purchase a peak flow meter to use at home. (They range from $15 to $30 on the Internet.) Repeat the test after Cycle 1 is complete. You will be surprised how much you can improve your lung function in such a short period of time.

Also, you can take this memory test before Day 1 and again on Day 18 to see just how quickly you can improve your short-term memory.

Memory Test

Test your short-term memory by looking at this grocery list for no more than 30 seconds. Then write down everything you can remember from the list on a piece of paper. See how many items you can remember. Then, perform the test again after you've completed Cycle 1 and see how much you've improved. You'll be surprised!

Spinach
Blueberries
Eggs
1 gallon of skim milk
Broccoli
Organic green beans
Baby carrots
4 chicken breasts
Oatmeal
Low-fat yogurt
Detergent
Whole pineapple
Walnuts

Before Beginning Cycle 1

Conduct a thorough cleaning of your living and work space (be sure to wear a dust mask while you're cleaning). This isn't about cleaning out your closet of clothes you don't wear; this is about removing dust and allergens. If you suffer from allergies, take your allergy medication a half hour before you begin the cleaning, and keep windows open for fresh air.

Why: This cleaning will give your respiratory system a bit of a break because you won't be breathing as many dust particles and pollens over the course of the 17 days.

General Guidelines for Cycle 1

1. Check the label on your daily multivitamin to make sure it includes these vitamins and dosages. If not, start taking supplements in conjunction with the multivitamin or simply replace your multivitamin with one that contains most of these amounts.

   - Vitamin C: 1,000 mg daily
   - Vitamin E: 200 IUs daily
   - Fish oil: 3 grams daily
   - B complex:

     Folic acid: .4 mg
     B-12: 2.4 mcg
     B-6: 1.3 mg

   - Selenium: .2 mg
   - Turmeric: 750 mg daily
   - Flaxseed oil: 1 tablespoon
   - Coenzyme Q10: 50 mg

2. Stop using perfume, hairspray, air freshener, and all aerosol cleaning products for this entire cycle. (Hey, a few bad hair days and smelly bathrooms are small prices to pay for getting your lungs working at their best!)

   Why: There are potentially toxic ingredients in these seemingly innocuous products that will interact negatively with other indoor pollutants (such as dust and animal dander). By taking a break from using these products, your lungs will enjoy a much-needed rest.

3. As you know, one of the anti-aging essentials is to stay hydrated, so let this serve as your reminder to drink at least six to eight 8-ounce glasses of water each day on this plan.

Tip: Get a reusable water bottle and keep it nearby all day, including when you're driving, working, etc. Depending on how many ounces it holds, you should be refilling it a few times daily.

4. Time how long you brush your teeth in the morning and at night by placing an egg timer next to the sink. Set it to two minutes—it's longer than you think, so keep brushing until the alarm goes off and floss afterward.

Reminder: People with the least amount of bacteria in their mouth and gums typically have better cognitive functioning than those with dirty mouths!

Restore: Cycle 1

You're all set to begin Restore! Some days include specific exercises, breathing techniques, or stretches shown in italics; you'll find these explained further in the Appendix.

DAY 1

Upon rising: Perform two sets of 15 *squat jacks*.

Within 30 minutes of waking: Eat a healthy breakfast including at least one item from the anti-inflammatory foods list and one cup of Thyme Tea (recipe on 47).

- *Ideas:* Spinach and egg-white omelet, fresh blueberries over oatmeal, pineapple chunks with Greek yogurt, pomegranate juice, and one whole egg.

Morning: Practice Dr. Mike's Meditation (found in Chapter 5) for 30 minutes. If possible, do this in a dark space by yourself.

Mid-morning: Call your doctor and make an appointment if:

- You're on medications and have any questions about the dosages, how many you're taking, and any new vitamins or supplements you're taking with them.
- You haven't had a doctor listen to your lungs in a year or more.
- You have any concerns about your heart, brain, or lung health.

Lunch: Include one vegetable high in carotenoids (dark leafy greens, carrots, tomatoes, watermelon, broccoli, squash, sweet potatoes).

Afternoon snack: six walnuts and one apple

Midday: Practice *Breath of Fire* for one minute. Take a break after 30 seconds, if necessary.

Late afternoon: Take a new route home from work or when you do errands today.

Evening: Perform two sets of one-minute *wall sits*.

Before dinner: Go on a 30-minute walk, jog, or run, depending on your fitness level.

- Alternatives: an at-home cardio DVD, gym class, or bike ride.

- Pick up the pace of your workout just a little every day this week to challenge your heart and lungs. Go a little farther or push yourself a little harder.

Dinner: Include at least two items from the anti-inflammatory foods list and sprinkle turmeric on these foods. (If you're taking turmeric supplements, there's no need to also put it in food.)

Before bed: Put four drops of essential oil in a pot of boiling water on the stove. Breathe in the scented steam for 10 minutes. (I like eucalyptus for this.)

DAY 2

Upon rising: Perform two sets of 30 *jumping jacks* and then perform a *standing chest expansion*.

Throughout the day: To help you become more aware of your breathing, concentrate on making your inhales and exhales match your footfalls when you're walking. And while sitting in the car or at a desk, concentrate on keeping both feet flat on the floor and your back straight so your chest is open. Take slow, deep breaths for 30 seconds, every hour.

Within 30 minutes of waking: Eat a healthy breakfast including at least one item from the anti-inflammatory foods list.

- *Idea:* Drink one glass of pomegranate juice or include pomegranate areoles in one cup of yogurt.

Morning: Practice Dr. Mike's Meditation for 30 minutes.

Midday: When you're in your car today, listen to a new radio station and different type of music.

Anytime: Experiment with ways to make drinking eight cups of water enjoyable.

- *Idea:* Put a few slices of cucumbers, strawberries, lemon, or orange in a refrigerated jug of water.

Mid-morning: If you regularly have trouble breathing or have any back/neck problems, consider asking your family practice doctor for a referral to a chiropractor.

Afternoon snack: Handful of blueberries, one apple, and a cup of Thyme Tea.

Evening: Perform two sets of 10 *lunges*.

Before dinner: Go on a 30-minute walk, jog, or run, depending on your fitness level.

- Alternatives: an at-home cardio DVD, gym class, or bike ride.
- Pick up the pace of your workout just a little every day this week to challenge your heart and lungs. Go a little farther or push yourself a little harder.

Dinner: Include at least two items from the anti-inflammatory foods list.

- *Idea:* Have pineapple slices for dessert. Or throw some pineapple chunks in the blender with low-fat coconut milk for a virgin anti-inflammatory piña colada!

Before Bed: Do a crossword puzzle.

- If you don't have time to complete it, just get it started and pick up where you left off later in this plan. (And you don't have to wait for the Sunday paper—there are lots of free crosswords online!)

DAY 3

Upon rising: Take your *resting heart rate*. Then, choose an upbeat song at least four minutes long and boogie down in your living room. Dance, jump, move, shake your body! Take your heart rate again. Did you get into your *cardio zone*?

Morning: Perform *cobra stretches*.

Within 30 minutes of waking: Eat a healthy breakfast including at least one item from the anti-inflammatory foods list.

• *Idea:* Salmon lox with whole-grain toast.

Mid-morning: Practice Dr. Mike's Meditation for 30 minutes.

Lunch: Include one vegetable high in carotenoids (dark leafy greens, asparagus, carrots, broccoli, citrus fruits, squash, sweet potatoes).

Midday: Practice saying simple phrases in another language for 15 minutes. Remember: Use it or lose it!

Afternoon snack: Eat one apple and either a handful of blueberries OR a smoothie with one cup low-fat coconut milk, blueberries, and one teaspoon agave nectar. (Note: You're going to be eating a lot of apples on this plan, so you may want to buy different types to keep it interesting.)

Late afternoon: Perform two sets of 15 *squats*.

Evening: Go surfing . . . Internet surfing!

• Spend 30 minutes on a search engine, looking up something you've always wanted to learn about, or planning an imaginary vacation to a faraway land!

Before dinner: Go on a 30-minute walk, jog, or run, depending on your fitness level.

• Alternatives: an at-home cardio DVD, gym class, or bike ride.

• Pick up the pace of your workout just a little every day this week to challenge your heart and lungs. Go a little farther or push yourself a little harder.

Dinner: Include at least two items from the anti-inflammatory foods list.

• *Idea:* Make an anti-inflammatory veggie feast by steaming broccoli, carrots, onions, and cauliflower, and add plenty of garlic.

DAY 4

Upon rising: Drop and give me 20 push-ups!

- Knees on the ground are okay, but try to work your way up to a regular push-up in the days ahead. Do as many as you can in a row, taking breaks if necessary. Ultimately, 20 is the goal.

All day: Concentrate on your posture. Do not hunch over! Let the oxygen flow deeper into your lungs by keeping your chest expanded.

Within 30 minutes of waking: Eat a healthy breakfast including at least one item from the anti-inflammatory foods list.

Morning: Practice Dr. Mike's Meditation for 30 minutes.

Lunch: Include an apple and one food high in polyunsaturated fat.

- *Idea:* Chop up your apple, and add a couple of walnuts and one teaspoon of sunflower seeds to the apple chunks.

Afternoon: Practice *straw breathing* to increase lung capacity.

Snack: One to two cups of steamed or raw broccoli.

- C'mon, you can do it. Spice it up with a salt-free mix like Mrs. Dash—kinda weird to recommend a specific brand since I don't do that elsewhere (or do it rarely, at least). Or pour some balsamic vinegar on top.

Late afternoon: Jump rope (your "rope" can be invisible) for two minutes.

Evening: Break out of your kitchen routine by rearranging your spice cabinet. Either alphabetize it or move everything on the right side to the left side so it's a little tougher to remember where everything is.

Before dinner: Go on a 30-minute walk, jog, or run, depending on your fitness level.

- *Alternatives:* an at-home cardio DVD, gym class, or bike ride.
- Pick up the pace of your workout just a little every day this week to challenge your heart and lungs. Go a little farther or push yourself a little harder.

Dinner: Include at least two items from the anti-inflammatory foods list and one vegetable high in carotenoids, and sprinkle turmeric on your vegetables.

DAY 5

Reminder: Have you been drinking eight cups of water throughout the day?

- Idea: Make ice cubes with berries, grapes, or other small pieces of fruit suspended in them.

Upon rising: Pretend that you're playing basketball for three minutes. Grab the invisible ball, then jump and shoot the ball. (Nobody is looking!)

- The point is to get your heart pumping, so really get your feet off the ground here and reach for that invisible basket.

Within 30 minutes of waking: Eat a healthy breakfast including at least one item from the anti-inflammatory foods list.

Mid-morning: Practice Dr. Mike's Meditation for 30 minutes.

Afternoon: Practice the *diaphragmatic breathing technique* for three minutes.

Afternoon snack: A handful of cherry tomatoes and one apple.

- *Idea:* Cut them up, mix them with vinegar and one teaspoon flaxseed oil, and add salt-free spices.
- *Alternative:* ¼ avocado.

Midday: Get your heart rate up by marching in place (get those knees HIGH!) for three minutes.

Before dinner: Go on a 30-minute walk, jog, or run, depending on your fitness level.

- *Alternatives:* an at-home cardio DVD, gym class, or bike ride.
- Pick up the pace of your workout just a little every day this week to challenge your heart and lungs. Go a little farther or push yourself a little harder.

Dinner: Include at least two items from the anti-inflammatory foods list.

Mid-evening: Solve a crossword puzzle or Sudoku puzzle, or play a game of any sort.

Before bed: Put four drops of essential oil in a pot of boiling water on the stove. Breathe in the scented steam for 10 minutes. (I like eucalyptus for this.)

DAY 6

Upon rising: Perform two sets of 10 *lunges*.

Within 30 minutes of waking: Eat a healthy breakfast including at least one item from the anti-inflammatory foods list and one cup of Thyme Tea.

Morning: Practice Dr. Mike's Meditation for 30 minutes.

Afternoon snack: A handful of raw baby carrots or chopped celery.

- *Idea:* Dip them in low-fat yogurt spiced up with dill, pepper, or other seasonings.

Midday: Practice *Breath of Fire* for one minute. Then, perform two sets of 20 *chair squats*.

Late afternoon: Practice saying simple phrases in another language for 15 minutes.

Before dinner: Go on a 30-minute walk, jog, or run, depending on your fitness level.

- *Alternatives:* an at-home cardio DVD, gym class, or bike ride.
- Pick up the pace of your workout just a little every day this week to challenge your heart and lungs. Go a little farther or push yourself a little harder.

Dinner: Include at least two items from the anti-inflammatory foods list and at least one vegetable high in carotenoids. Sprinkle turmeric on your vegetables.

Before bed: Brush your teeth with your nondominant hand. And don't forget the egg timer! Set it for two minutes.

DAY 7

Upon rising: Perform two sets of 15 *squat jacks*.

Within 30 minutes of waking: Eat a healthy breakfast including at least one item from the anti-inflammatory foods list.

Morning: Practice Dr. Mike's Meditation for 30 minutes.

Lunch: Include one vegetable high in carotenoids and one food high in polyunsaturated fat.

Afternoon snack: Eat six walnuts and one apple.

Midday: Practice *straw breathing* for two minutes.

Late afternoon: Perform two sets of one-minute *wall sits*.

Before dinner: Go on a 30-minute walk, jog, or run, depending on your fitness level.

- *Alternatives:* an at-home cardio DVD, gym class, or bike ride.
- Pick up the pace of your workout just a little every day this week to challenge your heart and lungs. Go a little farther or push yourself a little harder.

Dinner: Include at least two items from the anti-inflammatory foods list.

Evening: Play a card game you haven't played in a long time, or an online game.

DAY 8

Upon rising: Perform two sets of 50 *jumping jacks*.

Within 30 minutes of waking: Eat a healthy breakfast including at least one item from the anti-inflammatory foods list.

Morning: Practice Dr. Mike's Meditation for 30 minutes.

Morning: Take an extra-hot shower today and breathe the steam in deeply for two minutes to help keep your lungs clear.

Afternoon snack: A handful of mixed berries and one apple.

Midday: Jump rope (your "rope" can be invisible) for two minutes.

Before dinner: Go on a 30-minute walk, jog, or run, depending on your fitness level.

- *Alternatives:* an at-home cardio DVD, gym class, or bike ride.
- Pick up the pace of your workout just a little every day this week to challenge your heart and lungs. Go a little farther or push yourself a little harder.

Dinner: Include at least two items from the anti-inflammatory foods list.

Evening: Solve a crossword puzzle or Sudoku puzzle, or play a game of any sort.

DAY 9

Upon rising: First, take your *resting heart rate*. Then choose two upbeat songs for an approximate total of eight minutes, and boogie down in your living room. Get your heart pumping and see if you're in your *cardio zone*.

Within 30 minutes of waking: Eat a healthy breakfast including at least one item from the anti-inflammatory foods list and one apple.

Morning: Practice Dr. Mike's Meditation for 30 minutes.

Lunch: Include one vegetable high in carotenoids, but also taste a food you've never tried before.

- This should preferably be a vegetable or fruit.
- Other options are a type of fish, nut, or seed you've never tasted.

Midday: Perform the *diaphragmatic breathing exercise* for three minutes.

Afternoon snack: One cup chopped cucumber.

- *Idea:* Add dill weed, cracked pepper, balsamic vinegar, and flax-seed oil for flavor.

Anytime: Practice saying simple phrases in another language for 15 minutes.

Late afternoon: Get out your invisible basketball and practice your jump shot for two minutes.

- *Idea:* If volleyball is more your speed, practice spiking the ball over the net. The important thing here is that you're jumping!

Evening: While stopped at a stoplight, test your short-term memory and try memorizing the license plate on the car in front of you. See if you can recall it five minutes later.

Before dinner: Go on a 30-minute walk, jog, or run, depending on your fitness level.

- *Alternatives:* an at-home cardio DVD, gym class, or bike ride.
- Pick up the pace of your workout just a little every day this week to challenge your heart and lungs. Go a little farther or push yourself a little harder.

Dinner: Include at least two items from the anti-inflammatory foods list and sprinkle turmeric on your vegetables.

DAY 10

Upon rising: Have you been sipping plenty of water every day? Also, do *explosive lunges* for four minutes total. Then perform a *standing chest expansion* for two minutes.

Within 30 minutes of waking: Eat a healthy breakfast including at least one item from the anti-inflammatory foods list.

Morning: Practice Dr. Mike's Meditation for 30 minutes.

All day: Be conscious of your breathing. When sitting in the car or at a desk, concentrate on keeping both feet flat on the floor and your back straight. Take slow, deep breaths for 30 seconds, every hour.

Lunch: Include one vegetable high in carotenoids and one food high in polyunsaturated fat. Sprinkle turmeric on your vegetables.

Afternoon snack: A handful of blueberries and one apple.

Late afternoon: Perform two sets of one-minute *wall sits*.

Before dinner: Go on a 30-minute walk, jog, or run, depending on your fitness level.

- *Alternatives:* an at-home cardio DVD, gym class, or bike ride.
- Pick up the pace of your workout just a little every day this week to challenge your heart and lungs. Go a little farther or push yourself a little harder.

Dinner: Include at least two items from the anti-inflammatory foods list.

Evening: Solve a crossword puzzle or Sudoku puzzle, or play a game of any sort.

DAY 11

Upon rising: Drop and give me 20 pushups!

Within 30 minutes of waking: Eat a healthy breakfast including at least one item from the anti-inflammatory foods list and one cup of Thyme Tea.

Morning: Practice Dr. Mike's Meditation for 30 minutes.

Midmorning: Do some brain aerobics—while working on the computer today, try using your nondominant hand for controlling the mouse. It's challenging, but stick with it!

Lunch: Include one vegetable high in carotenoids.

Afternoon snack: A handful of walnuts and one apple.

Midday: Practice *Breath of Fire* for one minute.

Late afternoon: March in place at a fast pace for three minutes. Get those knees high! Is your heart pumping hard? Keep going for 10 minutes if you want an extra challenge.

Before dinner: Go on a 30-minute walk, jog, or run, depending on your fitness level.

- *Alternatives:* an at-home cardio DVD, gym class, or bike ride.

- Pick up the pace of your workout just a little every day this week to challenge your heart and lungs. Go a little farther or push yourself a little harder.

Dinner: Include at least two items from the anti-inflammatory foods list.

Evening: Go Internet surfing for 30 minutes. Learn about a different culture or country.

DAY 12

All day: Be more conscious of your calories and portions today, especially if you need to lose some weight. Try eating only half what is on your plate and put the fork down before you're full.

Upon rising: Jump up and down in place for two minutes. You don't have to get a lot of height for this to work. Then, perform *cobra stretches* for five minutes.

Within 30 minutes of waking: Eat a healthy breakfast including at least one item from the anti-inflammatory foods list and one apple.

Morning: Practice Dr. Mike's Meditation for 30 minutes.

Lunch: Include one vegetable high in carotenoids.

Anytime: Practice saying simple phrases in another language for 15 minutes.

Afternoon snack: One baked sweet potato. Just because it's called a sweet potato doesn't mean you should add sugar—try a sprinkle of cinnamon and one teaspoon of flaxseed oil.

Midday: Perform two sets of 10 *squats*. Rest for 10 minutes and then practice *straw breathing*.

Before dinner: Go on a 30-minute walk, jog, or run, depending on your fitness level.

- *Alternatives:* an at-home cardio DVD, gym class, or bike ride.
- Pick up the pace of your workout just a little every day this week to challenge your heart and lungs. Go a little farther or push yourself a little harder.

Dinner: Include at least two items from the anti-inflammatory foods list.

Evening: Give your brain a break from TV tonight. Awaken your brain cells by listening to classical music while reorganizing your sock or underwear drawer.

DAY 13

All day: Lighten up on your caloric intake today if you tend to be a heavy eater or if you're consuming more than 2,000 calories daily. Try eating only half what is on your plate, especially if you're trying to lose some weight.

Upon rising: Perform two sets of 15 *squat jacks*. Then, perform a *standing chest expansion* for two minutes.

Within 30 minutes of waking: Eat a healthy breakfast including at least one item from the anti-inflammatory foods list, one apple, and a cup of Thyme Tea.

Morning: Practice Dr. Mike's Meditation for 30 minutes.

Lunch: Include one vegetable high in carotenoids.

Afternoon snack: It's broccoli day again!

- Eat one to two cups of steamed (or raw) broccoli. Spice it up with a salt-free mix such as Mrs. Dash. Or pour some balsamic vinegar and one teaspoon flaxseed oil on top.

Midday: Turn on an upbeat playlist in your headphones and go on a brisk 10-minute walk OR "twist and shout" for a 10-minute mini dance party. (You may want to do this in private, or invite friends to join you!)

Before dinner: Go on a 30-minute walk, jog, or run, depending on your fitness level.

- *Alternatives:* an at-home cardio DVD, gym class, or bike ride.
- Pick up the pace of your workout just a little every day this week to challenge your heart and lungs. Go a little farther or push yourself a little harder.

Dinner: Include at least two items from the anti-inflammatory foods list.

Evening: Solve a crossword puzzle or Sudoku puzzle, or play a game of any sort.

DAY 14

Have you been drinking plenty of water? Keep it up!

Upon rising: Perform three sets of *planks*. Then, perform one minute of *cat/cow* stretches.

Within 30 minutes of waking: Eat a healthy breakfast including at least one item from the anti-inflammatory foods list and one apple.

Morning: Practice Dr. Mike's Meditation for 30 minutes.

Lunch: Include one vegetable high in carotenoids and one food high in polyunsaturated fat.

Mid-afternoon: Perform the *diaphragmatic breathing exercise* for three minutes.

Afternoon snack: Garlic green beans—steam some green beans with ½ chopped garlic clove. Or, sprinkle garlic powder on top. (You might want to have a breath mint ready!)

Late afternoon: Perform two sets of 20 *chair squats*.

Before dinner: Go on a 30-minute walk, jog, or run, depending on your fitness level.

- *Alternatives:* an at-home cardio DVD, gym class, or bike ride.

- Pick up the pace of your workout just a little every day this week to challenge your heart and lungs. Go a little farther or push yourself a little harder.

Dinner: Include at least two items from the anti-inflammatory foods list and sprinkle turmeric on your vegetables.

DAY 15

Upon rising: Perform two sets of 50 *jumping jacks* and two minutes of *standing chest expansion*.

Within 30 minutes of waking: Eat a healthy breakfast including at least one item from the anti-inflammatory foods list and one apple.

Morning: Practice Dr. Mike's Meditation for 30 minutes.

Mid-morning: Perform three minutes of *shadowboxing*.

Lunch: Include one vegetable high in carotenoids.

Afternoon: Practice *straw breathing* for two minutes. (Note: Is this getting easier for you?)

Afternoon snack: A handful of raw baby carrots or chopped celery.

Late afternoon: Practice saying simple phrases in another language for 15 minutes.

While driving: Try to memorize the license plate of the car in front of you. See if you can still remember it 10 minutes later.

Before dinner: Go on a 30-minute walk, jog, or run, depending on your fitness level.

- *Alternatives:* an at-home cardio DVD, gym class, or bike ride.
- Pick up the pace of your workout just a little every day this week to challenge your heart and lungs. Go a little farther or push yourself a little harder.

Dinner: Include at least two items from the anti-inflammatory foods list.

DAY 16

All day: Lighten up on your caloric intake today. Try eating only half of what is on your plate.

Upon rising: Drop and give me 20 pushups! Then, perform *cobra stretches* for five minutes.

Within 30 minutes of waking: Eat a healthy breakfast including at least one item from the anti-inflammatory foods list.

Mid-morning: Practice Dr. Mike's Meditation for 30 minutes.

Lunch: Include one vegetable high in carotenoids.

Afternoon snack: A handful of pomegranate areoles, or a handful of blueberries and one apple.

Late afternoon: Practice *Breath of Fire* for one minute. Then, perform two sets of 50 *jumping jacks*.

Before dinner: Go on a 30-minute walk, jog, or run, depending on your fitness level.

- *Alternatives:* an at-home cardio DVD, gym class, or bike ride.
- Pick up the pace of your workout just a little every day this week to challenge your heart and lungs. Go a little farther or push yourself a little harder.

Dinner: Include at least two items from the anti-inflammatory foods list.

Evening: Solve a crossword puzzle or Sudoku puzzle, or play a game of any sort.

DAY 17

Upon rising: Drop and give me 20 push-ups! How many can you do in a row now?

Within 30 minutes of waking: Eat a healthy breakfast including at least one item from the anti-inflammatory foods list and one apple, plus one cup of Thyme Tea.

Mid-morning: Practice Dr. Mike's Meditation for 30 minutes.

Throughout the day: While you're walking, concentrate on making your inhales and exhales match your footfalls. You should naturally be more conscious of your breath by now.

Mid-morning: Practice *Breath of Fire* for one minute.

Lunch: Include one vegetable high in carotenoids and sprinkle turmeric on your meal.

Afternoon snack: A handful of cherry tomatoes.

- Feel free to cut them up, mix them with vinegar, and add salt-free spices.
- *Alternative:* ¼ avocado.

Midday: Perform two sets of one-minute *wall sits*.

Evening: Break out of your routine by taking a new route home from work or when you do errands today.

Before dinner: Go on a 30-minute walk, jog, or run, depending on your fitness level.

- *Alternatives:* an at-home cardio DVD, gym class, or bike ride.
- Pick up the pace of your workout just a little every day this week to challenge your heart and lungs. Go a little farther or push yourself a little harder.

Dinner: Include at least two items from the anti-inflammatory foods list and one food high in polyunsaturated fat.

Congratulations! You completed the Restore Cycle. Beyond feeling great, you can actually see the tangible results of the improvements made by completing the optional bonuses we discussed. Compare your cholesterol and CRP levels from before Cycle 1 to after just 17 short days. Now imagine the improvements you can make when you continue making these simple efforts.

Remember that memory test from the beginning of the Cycle? See how far your short-term memory came by looking at this grocery list for no more than 30 seconds, then writing down what you can remember. I'm willing to bet you can remember a list a lot longer than this one! Ready? Set. Go.

Grocery List for Memory Test

Frozen broccoli
Skim milk

Oatmeal
Strawberries
Zucchini
Carrots
Fresh flowers
Lean ground turkey
Raspberries
Cottage cheese
Mangoes
Almonds
Vitamin C supplements

By the end of the Restore Cycle, you should be feeling fantastic overall. You're breathing with more ease, thinking more clearly, feeling energetic, and probably even fitting into your clothes better. Your circulatory, respiratory, and nervous systems respond so quickly to such minor efforts and subtle changes, and in just these 17 days you actually took huge strides toward delaying—even reversing—the five factors of aging. See how easy it can be to control those factors? You've just built the groundwork for balancing methylation; preventing heart, lung, and nervous system impairment; avoiding cellular glycation and thus keeping your organs flexible; halting oxidative stress, and putting out the fires of inflammation. All that just by some simple lifestyle tweaks. Pretty amazing stuff, huh?

This is only the beginning . . . follow me for more simple changes you can make to your everyday routine to further preserve the health of all your body's systems. Now that we've started the transformation within your heart, lungs, and brain, we'll turn our focus toward your immune, digestive, endocrine, and musculoskeletal systems. These are your supportive systems, the ones that protect, nourish, and regulate you and give you the ability to move. It's time to rebuild and vitalize them so you can enjoy great health and vigor as you make your way toward your 100th birthday. Let's continue!

PART THREE

• •

Cycle 2: Rebuild

I want you to be glowing with health, bursting with energy, and looking and feeling as fabulous as you possibly can—which is the point of Cycle 2: Rebuild. It focuses on immunity, digestion, hormonal health, and body strength and fitness. As we get older, certain things happen to these secondary (but super-vital) parts of our bodies. Your body becomes less able to resist some diseases as the immune system begins to weaken in midlife. Digestion slows down. Your body slackens its ability to process blood sugar. Wear and tear can lead to arthritic joints. Muscle tissue decreases and you begin to lose those attractive contours of your youth.

You'll begin to reverse all those ravages of time in Cycle 2. I'll show you how to bolster your immune system so you're rarely sick—which means no downtime and more fun in life. I'll talk about how to protect your digestive system from unhealthy slowdowns so that you feel energetic every day. There's a lot you can do, too, to prevent hormonal conditions like diabetes. We'll talk about how. Then I switch the focus to your bones and muscles, and how to get them as fit and strong as possible. You definitely don't want to be among the unfit! They're three times more likely to die prematurely than their fit peers. Remember, you want to live to 100 and beyond—and stay healthy and fit. It's not that difficult, either. You only need make a few lifestyle tweaks. But they all add up to a fitter, more attractive, and more vibrant you. So what are those tweaks? Keep turning the pages and you'll find out.

CHAPTER 7

Your Body's Guard

When your immune system goes on the fritz, you're susceptible to three things: infections, autoimmune disease, and cancer (not to mention just being cranky because nobody likes being sick!). To understand why, and learn how to protect yourself, let me show you how immune cells work. Once you get the lay of the land, my advice for keeping your immune system in tip-top shape will make more sense, and you'll be well on your way to living 100 happy, healthy years if you just follow my 17 Day Plan.

Immune System 101

Every day, your body is under assault from germs and other bad guys, whether they come from the mucus spray of your child's sneeze, the coughing co-worker in the cubicle next to you, or even the pathogens you could be encountering simply by crossing the street. Fortunately, the body contains various types of immune cells to protect you. Some of these cells recognize the invaders, others send out warnings throughout your body about the invasion, another type gobbles them right up, and still others act as reinforcements. Together, they really do function much like an army, each type with its different jobs.

The immune system is more complicated than you may think. There are two major elements: the innate immune system and the adaptive immune system. And no surprise here: Your immune system, on the whole, evolves as you get older.

Innate immunity functions like the castle walls, and even a moat, to keep germs from entering the body. Your skin, your cough reflex, the mucous membranes in your nose, even the stomach acid in your digestive system all act as blockades to stop the viral, bacterial, or other types of invaders. Next, just in case there are surviving pathogens, your body has a special set of cells that go into action. These immune cells include:

T-cells. Essentially, T-cells are a type of white blood cell that your body uses to target and kill foreign cells such as viruses or bacteria. What's really cool about these guys is that once you've had an infection, they program themselves to kill that specific pathogen if they encounter it again. They stay in your body for a long time, always on the lookout for a foreign threat. They're like little snipers protecting you! You probably have heard about T-cells in relation to someone with HIV or AIDS. That's because someone with this condition no longer has enough T-cells to fight off infections.

Macrophages. These cells are like the neighborhood watch—they police your body, constantly on the lookout for potentially dangerous tissue or cells that they can kill. When they find an invader, they just gobble it up! They have deadly chemicals that destroy the enemy while they're ingesting it. However, as we get older, our macrophages slow down their patrol. Since one type of foreign cells they kill is cancer, this may explain why we're more likely to get cancer when we're older. The point is, we want to do what we can to keep our macrophages functioning well.

Now let's move on to your adaptive immune system. It's a lot more involved because it's made up of many different organs. When you get swollen glands on your neck because you have strep throat, those glands are part of your lymphatic system, which plays a big role in your immunity. If you've ever had a sore throat or a cold, your doctor probably felt around on your neck to check out your lymph nodes. And if your lymph nodes were swollen, that's because they were filling up with extra fluid called lymph to fight an infection going on in your body. Lymph is essentially made up of a mixture of infection-fighting white blood cells and a white or clear liquid (chyle) that originates in your small intestine. Think of your lymph system as a network of filters that extends all over your body. The lymph moves around, picking up infectious invaders and destroying them within your nodes. The lymph nodes are positioned in groups in several key areas of your body: your neck, groin, armpits, abdomen, and chest. Other organs within your lymph system are the thymus, spleen, bone marrow, adenoids, and tonsils. We'll talk more about this key system, and how to keep it healthy, a little later in this chapter.

Sometimes the immune system goes awry. That happens when immune cells get confused and think healthy cells and other tissues are really the enemy. They attack perfectly healthy cells in a sort of friendly fire known as an autoimmune disease. For example, when the immune system attacks the hair follicles, the result can be complete baldness, known medically as alopecia areata. Or immune cells might attack healthy cells in your joints, causing rheumatoid arthritis.

In cases like these, the body has to get its story straight. To do that, it needs the right resources. That's where lifestyle choices come into play—diet, exercise, stress management, and other tools. If you can fortify your immune system, you'll likely get sick less often, potentially avoiding everything from the common cold to cancer. Less sickness means a long, healthy, and productive life . . . hopefully 100 happy, healthy years.

LYMPH DRAINAGE MASSAGE

Whether you simply want your facial skin to look revitalized or you're desperate to keep your allergies at bay, you should consider learning how to perform a face massage on yourself because it encourages drainage of your lymph. It's smart to do this right before you wash your face at night. Starting toward the center of your forehead, gently press your fingers against the skin and move in circles. Stay there for three to five seconds and then move on to your outer forehead, and then down to your temples. Move inward toward your nose, but not directly under your eyes. Continue with the circular movements, down your cheeks to the outside of your mouth. Next, you'll focus on your jaw area, just in front of your ears and down to your neck. Be very gentle in this area. Finish the massage with very gentle downward strokes starting from the outside of your face and moving down to your neck. I also recommend this for when you have a cold or sinus infection, because it can help with the sinus pressure you feel. It can also stimulate your lymph system to work a little harder in your favor.

How Your Immune System Ages

Like the other systems we've talked about, your immune system ages in some not-so-pleasant ways:

Inflammation ramps up with age. That means we're more susceptible to heart disease, arthritis, frailty, type 2 diabetes, physical disability, and dementia, among other problems.

Fewer antibodies. Antibodies are produced by the immune system when an antigen is spotted in the vicinity. Antigens are large molecules that sit on the surface of cells, viruses, fungi, bacteria, and some nonliving matter such as toxins, chemicals, and foreign particles. With age, the number of antibodies produced in response to an antigen diminishes, making it harder for your body to fight off infection.

Compromised immune cells. As you get older, you have to work a little harder to maintain a healthy immune system. That's because your body naturally creates a lower number of T-cells, which also affects how your body responds to vaccines. For example, let's say you got the flu shot this year. The reason flu shots work is because your T-cells (the ones that aren't already programmed to fight some other invader) will grab on to that vaccine and produce an immune response in your body so that strain of the flu can't infect you. But if you have fewer T-cells, this process doesn't work quite as well. (Of course there are exceptions to every rule, such as the shingles vaccine, which can be very effective in older people who've already had the chicken pox virus when they were younger.)

One more thing: As your body's clock ticks away, you're probably not going to produce as many white blood cells as you did when you were a kid. Thus, your defenses are a little weaker than they once were.

Autoimmune problems. If your immune system can't correctly target alien cells in the body, then you can get an autoimmune or immune-suppressed disease like celiac disease, psoriasis, lupus, Lyme disease, rheumatoid arthritis, or irritable bowel syndrome. These diseases are the result of the weird "friendly fire" taking place in your immune system. Autoimmune disease can affect people of any age, but we are at an increased risk for developing them as we grow older.

Lymphedema. If your lymphatic system isn't functioning properly as you age, your lymph can pool up, causing visible swelling in your legs and sometimes arms. This can be a result of a blockage or obstruction within your lymph nodes.

Cancer risk. When your own cells turn into foreign invaders in your body, you can develop cancer. Under normal conditions, your body purposely shuts some cells down in a process called apoptosis—which basically means that cells commit suicide. Apoptosis goes on continually in your body after normal cells have done their jobs. More specifically, apoptosis is about making sure the right cells shut down and the necessary cells don't. If the wrong brain cells shut down, you can develop dementia. If the wrong heart cells shut down, you can get heart disease. And if a cell that is harmful doesn't kill itself off as it should—if it loses its apoptotic capabilities—cancer can invade. Cancer cells are renegade cells that don't kill themselves. The key for you is to strengthen your immune system so it can find those cancerous cells and take them out. That's why the strategies I've outlined below are so important.

SUPPLEMENTS THAT SUPPORT YOUR IMMUNE SYSTEM

- **Zinc:** 11 mg total daily for men and 8 mg total daily for women
- **Vitamin C:** 1,000 mg total daily
- **Folic acid:** 400 mcg total daily
- **Ginseng:** As directed

Why? Zinc, vitamin C, and folic acid all strengthen the immune system so it can better defend you against colds and all types of infections. Check the label of your multivitamin to see if the appropriate dosages are included, and if not, take them separately.

One more supplement to consider, but to use within reason, is ginseng. There have been conflicting reports over the years about its usefulness, but some of the most compelling research shows that it can be very beneficial to people suffering from chronic illnesses. As always, discuss supplements and their side effects with your doctor, but you should consider making this part of your regimen.

DO WHAT WITH ALGAE?

Spirulina is a type of blue-green algae that might help support your body's immunity. Further testing is needed to prove this, but I do think it's worth trying. The Aztecs of Mexico certainly believed in it; they dried it in the sun and supplemented their diet with it regularly. Spirulina is made up of 62 percent amino acids, and it's a rich source of protein, B-12, and beta carotene.

Now, I don't buy into any of the "superfood" hype, and I'm a huge believer in getting back to the basics. But spirulina is loaded with nutrients, so it probably can't hurt to incorporate it in moderation. Always consult your doctor before adding supplements like spirulina, and it shouldn't be mixed with immunosuppressants.

The Number-One Strategy: Fight Glycation

As I explained in chapter 1, glycation is a harmful process in the body in which sugar molecules bind to proteins or fats. This linkage produces advanced glycation end-products, which attack virtually every part of the body, and they tend to aggravate immune cells. AGEs are one of the leading causes of deterioration in many organs. They bring on inflammation and increased free radical production, both of which are at the core of aging.

If glycation is so damaging, will cutting down on sources of sugar get us on the road to living 100 happy, healthy years? I believe so. Here's why: Glycation alters the structure of protein in the body. That altered protein gets recognized by the immune system as foreign, so it is then susceptible to an autoimmune attack. Remember, that's the "friendly fire" situation in which your body mistakenly thinks its own substances, tissues, or organs are the enemy, so it attacks them. Moreover, glycated proteins have been implicated in heart disease, in the end-organ damage seen in diabetics, and in kidney failure, nerve damage, diabetes, cataracts, and even cancer. Have I made a strong enough case here? Because glycation is implicated in these life-shortening conditions, it's critical that you take measures to reduce it as much as possible—if, that is, you'd like to stay healthy for decades to come.

So what can you do? Reducing the amount of sugar you eat, particularly high fructose corn syrup, is an important step toward minimizing the amount of glycation that occurs in the body. The research is pretty clear on this recommendation. Taking in excess fructose (as you'd do from drinking large soft drinks daily or eating lots of sugary foods regularly) overwhelms your body's fructose-metabolizing capacity. As a result, excess fructose spills into the bloodstream. That excess can aggravate autoimmune reactions, increase inflammation, and in general, accelerate aging. So toss the sugary drinks and snacks and find healthy, sugar-free options instead. Some easy replacements include fresh juices, sugar-free beverages, fresh fruits, nuts, raw veggies, low-fat dairy, and whole grains.

Supportive Strategies

Wash your hands. A lot of infections are passed by hand—almost all infections, actually, especially during flu season. You might hear your spouse coughing and you think, "Great, now I'm going to catch a cold, too." But, it's the germs on surfaces, not the germs in the air, that you catch more easily. Here's an example: Suppose you're traveling. The person in front of you with the flu touches the escalator handrail (one of the most germ-infested surfaces known to man). Now everyone who touches the escalator gets those germs on their hands, and the next time they touch their mouth, those germs have found a way into their body. So, it's important to wash your hands habitually: before meals, after you go to the bathroom, after every handshake, and after you touch anything in public places. (No, I'm not trying to instill a fear of shaking people's hands! I simply want you to take germs seriously.)

Keep the bacteria in your gut healthy. Your digestive system may not be the first thing you think of when you envision your immune system at work. But the bacterial balance in your stomach and intestines plays a huge role in your ability to ward off illness. (I told you everything was connected in ways you never knew!) You have 100 trillion bacteria in your belly, ten times the number of cells in your body, and some of those bacterial species can be deadly. So you need to make sure you have enough of the good bacteria to ward off the bad. Probiotics can help you strike the healthy balance you need. Essentially, probiotics are "friendly" bacteria that provide many health benefits, in addition to boosting immunity. They can aid digestion, improve nutrient absorption, and even help with weight loss.

Normally classified as dietary supplements, probiotics are found in foods such as kefir and yogurt. So beneficial are probiotics that other foods are being fortified with them. There's even a probiotic whole-grain cereal, Kashi Vive, that you can eat to capitalize on these healthful bacteria. Or simply take a probiotic supplement daily, such as Culturelle or Align. Probiotics help strike the healthy balance you need.

Eat natural, "whole" foods. A diet rich in whole foods is one that's packed with foods that are very close to their natural, unprocessed and unrefined form. The closer the food is to nature, the better it is for your immunity. Load up on veggies, such as carrots, sweet potatoes, onions, celery, broccoli, cauliflower, and all the leafy greens, and all fruits, because they contain antioxidants like vitamin C and beta-carotene that your immunity "army" needs to fight off infections. And you should eat them as close to their natural state as possible. That means either raw or lightly steamed. (It's not "bad" to sauté or roast them, but raw or lightly steamed, the vegetables are more nutrient-dense.) If you find vegetables bland, season them with herbs, throw them in smoothies, or hide them in pureed soups. Make it your personal mission to become a veggie fanatic. It doesn't always have to be a boring salad. Get creative! (See my Mashed Un-Potatoes recipe for inspiration!)

Dr. Mike's Mashed Un-Potatoes

Vegetables, especially ones high in antioxidants, are great protectors of your immunity. And I am willing to bet that once you taste these, you'll never go back to regular mashed potatoes because you won't miss the butter, sour cream, and loads of salt that often go into making mashed potatoes so delicious. Plus, cauliflower is super-high in the antioxidant vitamin C. It also has folate (which is in the vitamin B family) and potassium. Trust me on this; just try it!

1 head white cauliflower
Water for steaming
Salt-free spices
Pepper to taste
Optional: Wasabi paste

Chop up the cauliflower into chunks, and steam until it's soft.

Place the chunks into a food processor or blender.

Blend it until it's smooth, adding in your favorite salt-free spices, such as garlic or Italian seasoning (or wasabi paste for a kick) and pepper.

Continue tasting it as you add spices.

Serve and enjoy!

Embrace berries. While I'm on the topic of antioxidants, I'd like to take a moment to sing the praises of berries. Strawberries, blueberries, blackberries, raspberries, and the like are all sweet, delicious little immunity powerhouses. They are loaded with various antioxidants, including vitamin C. Put them on top of oatmeal or in a low-fat smoothie, or eat a handful as a snack.

Delete "white" foods from your diet. I always tell my patients: With the exceptions of cauliflower and low-fat yogurts or cheeses, there are very few white foods that are healthy for you. I'm referring to simple sugars, refined carbohydrates, foods that have been stripped of their natural nutrients and fiber, such as the white flour in many baked goods, white pasta (versus whole wheat), white rice, and, of course, white sugar—they're just empty calories with zero nutritional value. Even in moderation, they'll make you feel—and look—old before your time. In terms of your immunity, simple carbohydrates, such as the ones found in candy, cause your blood sugars to spike after you eat them. When that happens, the excessive glucose essentially gets crowded in your blood and affects your circulation. Anytime your circulation is affected, that means your blood can't get to a problem as quickly. And if your blood can't get there, of course, your white blood cells can't get there either, which leaves your body unable to heal itself or fight off infection vigorously. Rule of thumb: if it's white, get it out of sight!

Eat foods high in selenium. Selenium, a trace mineral found in certain foods, is essential to a properly functioning immune system and a deficiency can compromise your overall immunity. This mineral is a constituent of glutathione, a powerful antioxidant and immune booster made naturally by your body. Selenium helps break down hydrogen peroxide—one of the most harmful free radicals around—into water. Mounds of research show that selenium can help fight infections, maintain brain function as we get older, and prevent some cancers. You need to get enough selenium in your diet, but you shouldn't go overboard, because too much selenium can cause other health issues. Be sure to consume moderate amounts of lean meats, some seafood such as tuna and cod, sunflower seeds, or eggs. A single Brazil nut contains all the selenium you need for a day, so instead of worrying about supplemental selenium, snack on one of these delicious nuts each day.

Venture outdoors. Vitamin D, which your body naturally produces when you're exposed to sunlight, also offers some major support to your immunity. One study at the University of Copenhagen showed that vitamin D can actually trigger your immune cells to go into action. It also indicated that if you don't have enough vitamin D, your T-cells can't react properly to infection. So, go outside and soak up a few rays. (Be careful not to burn, though! Just 10 to 15 minutes daily in the sunshine is all you really need.)

Get quality shut-eye. Getting enough good sleep on a regular basis is imperative to maintaining healthy immunity. I know you can't always have a perfect night's sleep, so don't beat yourself up if you work round the clock one night or stay out later than you should. But keep in mind that even one lousy night of sleep has been shown to increase inflammation in your body and could increase your risk for autoimmune diseases. So no more *Mad Men* reruns late at night; your sleep is more important!

Take two baby aspirin every day. Taking aspirin every day may cut your risk of many cancers and prevent tumors from spreading, according to some promising new research. This humble painkiller works by curbing chronic inflammation in your body, which is at the root of some cancers. A study published in *The Lancet*, a medical journal, found that daily use of aspirin over several years can trim the risk of some cancers by as much as 75 percent. Daily aspirin use may also reduce the risk of cancer spreading (metastatic disease), particularly in patients with colorectal cancer. Your best bet is to take two baby aspirin every day. As always, check with your doctor before beginning this, or any drug regimen, as it can have negative side effects, especially if you have stomach ulcers.

The Anti-Aging Essentials and Your Immune System

#1: Movement. Moving your body boosts your immune system by increasing your circulation. Remember what I said about how sugary foods impede your circulation, which means white blood cells can't address a foreign invader fast enough? Well, exercise does just the opposite; it gets your heart and blood pumping so that your white blood cells and other immune cells can get where they need to go.

#2: Maintain a healthy weight. Overweight people tend to suffer from more infections and illnesses, and while studies haven't identified the exact reason why, they have shown that overweight or obese people's immune cells don't respond adequately to invaders of all types. But don't fear—you'll find some simple tips you can apply right away to lose weight in a hurry.

#3: Stay hydrated. This maintains the mucous membranes in your nose and lungs, which makes it harder for viruses or bacteria to latch on and make you sick.

#4: Quit smoking. Did you know smokers take more sick days from work than nonsmokers? They're more likely to get colds, the flu, and other illnesses because their immune systems are putting in overtime to clear out all the toxins coming in from the smoke. Unfortunately, the same is true in terms of their increased risk for all types of cancer, coronary artery disease, emphysema, bronchitis—the list is a mile long. But as soon as you quit, your immunity starts to improve right away.

#5: *Supplement*. Above, you'll find information on the best supplements to improve the function of your immune system.

Check out the Appendix for ideas, resources, and recommendations for how to implement all five of these anti-aging essentials. You'll also find some ideas within the Cycle 2: Rebuild 17 Day Plan.

IF YOU NEED TO DROP SOME POUNDS . . .

If you're obese, your immune cells and your lymph system don't function properly. I suggest that you talk to your doc about getting on a 1,200- to 1,500-calorie-a-day diet to lose weight. Dieting isn't easy, so let me give you a few practical ways to shed some weight or keep your weight under control—these are very low in effort and very high in rewards. Here it goes:

- **Don't stuff yourself.** Just eat until you're satisfied. Overeating is one of the biggest reasons for weight gain. Push yourself away from the table before that uncomfortable feeling sets in.

- **Eat smaller portions.** To get the knack of this, buy calorie-controlled foods for awhile, either from the grocery freezer case or from a diet delivery service if your budget permits. The allotted portions will give you an idea of how much (or how little) you need to eat for weight loss. You'll be amazed that it doesn't take truckloads of food to satisfy your appetite.

- **Make simple calorie swaps.** Trade in premium high-fat ice cream for low-fat frozen yogurt, for example. You'll save about 100 calories automatically. Spread mustard on your sandwiches rather than mayonnaise for another 100-calorie cut. Shun fried chicken and go for baked chicken with a little seasoning, and save 200 to 300 calories. Say "no" to sugary sodas and have water instead. Every soda you don't drink saves 150 calories. If you make all three swaps in one day, you'll cut nearly 500 calories from your diet.

- **Always eat breakfast.** Dieters who start the day with a healthy meal lose more weight than breakfast skippers; that's a known fact. Have an egg or two, a slice of whole-wheat toast, and a fresh fruit; or a bowl of whole-grain cereal with yogurt and fresh fruit. Meals like these will keep you energized and protect you from overeating later on.

- **Get rid of junk food.** Clear your kitchen, car, and office of processed food. Remember, "Out of sight, out of mind." You can't eat it if it's not there.

LAUGH LONGER TO LIVE LONGER

You've heard the saying that "laughter is the best medicine." Here's one reason why it's true: A good belly laugh greatly increases the amount of oxygen you're taking in. This, in turn, nourishes and energizes important organs like your heart and lungs. Furthermore, a giggle has been shown to enhance your immune system by encouraging production of antibodies and T-cells. Researchers have observed this phenomenon by analyzing blood samples in experiments designed to provoke laughter in volunteers. We aren't sure how this happens, but it's definitely a part of the mind-body connection in health and longevity.

Laughter can even relieve pain with the natural endorphin release it causes. One more thing (although I could go on all day): Experts at the University of Maryland found that your blood vessels react differently when you watch a comedy of some kind as opposed to a drama. Study participants who watched comedies (and therefore laughed) experienced normal blood flow through the vessels, while people who watched dramas experienced impeded blood flow. The lesson? Laughter improves circulation, which in turn boosts immunity.

It may feel silly, but "laughter yoga" is a big trend these days for good reason. Just take 10 minutes to think of something hilarious, or watch a funny YouTube video.

Before you start the Cycle 2: 17-Day Plan, take this quiz and score yourself. Then, take the quiz again after you've completed the plan. Your results might just surprise you!

Is Your Immune System on Its Way to 100 Happy, Healthy Years?

1. **How often do you get sick with a cold or flu, on average?**

    A. More than twice a year □ 0 points

    B. Maybe just once a year □ 2 points

    C. Never □ 4 points

2. **How often do members of your family get sick?**

    A. Frequently; someone is always running to the doctor. □ 0 points

    B. Sometimes; we make trips to the doctor at least once a month.
       □ 2 points

    C. Hardly ever; everyone is pretty healthy. □ 4 points

3. **How often do you laugh out loud?**

   A. I can't remember the last time I laughed. ☐ 0 points

   B. I laugh a few times per week. ☐ 2 points

   C. I find something to laugh about on a daily basis. ☐ 4 points

4. **How much sleep have you been getting in recent weeks?**

   A. Five hours per night or less ☐ 0 points

   B. Nine or more hours per night ☐ 2 points

   C. Six to eight hours per night ☐ 4 points

5. **How would you rate your stress level?**

   A. Very high; I feel stressed most of the time. ☐ 0 points

   B. High; I experience stress a few days a week. ☐ 1 point

   C. Moderate; I am stressed out at least once a week. ☐ 2 points

   D. Low; I don't get stressed easily. ☐ 4 points

6. **Your diet mainly includes:**

   A. A lot of junk: fried foods, sodas, fast foods, and processed (packaged) foods ☐ 0 points

   B. Carbohydrates like pizza, white bread, pastas, and sweets, along with some protein, including red meat ☐ 1 point

   C. Lots of vegetables, fruits, whole grains, chicken, and fish ☐ 4 points

7. **Do you take antioxidant supplements?**

   A. No, I hate pills. ☐ 0 points

   B. Only when I remember, which is rare ☐ 1 point

   C. Yes, I take them daily. ☐ 4 points

8. **Do you smoke?**

   A. Yes, regularly. ☐ 0 points

   B. I quit within the last year. ☐ 1 point

   C. I gave it up five or more years ago ☐ 2 points

   D. I have never smoked. ☐ 4 points

9. **How often do you wash your hands?**

   A. I am really bad about it and rarely wash my hands. ☐ 0 points

   B. I wash my hands once per day, on average. ☐ 1 point

C. I wash my hands only after I go to the bathroom. ☐ 2 points

D. I wash my hands frequently throughout the day. ☐ 4 points

---

10. **How much time do you spend outside?**

    A. Only as long as it takes me to walk to my car ☐ 0 points

    B. About 10 to 15 minutes total per week ☐ 1 point

    C. I'm outside at least 10 minutes daily. ☐ 4 points

---

11. **If you're overweight, are you currently using a healthy method to lose the weight?**

    A. No ☐ 0 points

    B. Yes ☐ 4 points

    C. I'm not overweight. ☐ 4 points

---

12. **How do you generally feel?**

    A. I'm always tired, achy, or feeling run down. ☐ 0 points

    B. I feel okay, but I rarely feel great. ☐ 2 points

    C. I feel great most of the time and have plenty of energy. ☐ 4 points

---

13. **Do you take probiotics regularly?**

    A. No ☐ 0 points   B. Yes ☐ 4 points

---

14. **Are members of your family, including your grandparents, long-lived (85+ years)?**

    A. No ☐ 0   B. Yes ☐ 4

Scoring:

0–11: URGENT; if you get sick all the time and constantly feel run down, see your doctor about the current state of your immune system.

12–22: DANGEROUS; make some immediate changes to bolster your immunity.

23–33: MODERATELY RISKY; start incorporating my suggestions into your routines.

34–44: AVERAGE; you have room for additional change.

45–56: EXCELLENT; stay on this positive course.

Your body has been equipped with some very high-tech defense systems, but they do require care and attention. Follow the suggestions in this chapter, and you'll give your immune system a fighting chance to protect you from harm. The less illness that invades your body over a lifetime, the longer your lifetime could last *and* the more you'll be able to enjoy it!

CHAPTER 8

Listen to Your Gut

I see a lot of digestive problems in my private practice. No surprise, considering that every year approximately 70 million adults in America suffer from tummy troubles such as diarrhea, abdominal pain, constipation, and numerous other symptoms that cause discomfort or worse. Poor digestion can also be at the root of a bunch of other problems such as fatigue, skin rashes, headaches, poor concentration, and moodiness—symptoms you wouldn't think had anything to do with digestion.

And it's not as though you can just avoid food to make the problems go away, right? Aside from needing food to live, food is a national obsession! Doesn't it seem as if our lives revolve around it? We're perpetually planning the next meal. The first date is always over dinner. From the Thanksgiving feast to Fourth of July cookouts, every holiday we celebrate boils down to sitting around a table and stuffing ourselves. While I do hope your eating habits will have changed by the time you finish reading this book (or sooner!), I'm certainly not able to change the fact that food plays a central role in our lives. So let's keep your digestive system healthy!

The information within this chapter will help you lower your chances of suffering from dangerous digestive diseases and enjoy good gut health well into old age. Doctor's orders: Get serious about your digestive health. The first step is to gain a basic understanding of the structures and functions involved in digestion. Shall we begin?

Digestive System 101

Put simply, digestion is your body's process of extracting the necessary nutrients and energy from the food you eat. And the process begins even before you put one morsel into your mouth—just smelling something like bacon sizzling in the pan, or chocolate chip cookies emerging from

the oven, starts your digestion. You may even be salivating just thinking about it! That saliva is the first step. Once you do eat, saliva breaks
down the food a little, along with chewing, both of which make it possible for you to swallow the food. Your tongue gets into the act, too, by
pushing the food toward your esophagus. The main job of your esophagus is to move the food down to the next stop on the path, which is your
stomach. Next, your stomach uses powerful gastric juices to take that
food from a solid to a liquid to make the work easier for your small intestines.

Stretched from end to end, your small intestines are between 15 and
20 feet long. This is where a lot of the magic happens. The small intestines work in concert with the pancreas, gallbladder, and liver to help
your body soak up all the proteins, fats, minerals, vitamins, water, and
other vital nutrients from the food you ate.

Next, and this step is key, the nutrients provided by your meal pass
from the intestine right into your bloodstream. This nutrient-rich blood
goes directly to the liver for processing. The liver filters out toxins and
wastes, and turns some of the waste into bile. The liver even helps calculate how many nutrients will go to the rest of the body, and how many
will go into storage. For example, the liver stores vitamin A, vitamin D,
and glycogen, a type of sugar the body uses for energy.

Everything that's left from your meal that the body doesn't need is
considered waste. This waste travels to the large intestine, which then
pushes the feces into the rectum. The rectum is the very last stop on the
digestive tract. The waste stays there until you feel the urge to go to the
bathroom. I think you know the rest!

But let's rewind to the large intestine for a moment. It is here that
you'll find a huge colony of living, friendly microflora (probiotics), which
play a key role in digestive health. Intestinal microflora help fight cancer,
produce vitamins, degrade bile, promote immunity, and digest nutrients.
These friendly bacteria generally outnumber bad bacteria. However, if you
eat too much junk food, stress out a lot, take antibiotics often, or have
infections, that balance can be easily lost. Bad bacteria start outnumber-
ing and overwhelming the friendly bacteria, compromising your digestive health. Really, the large intestine is the biggest immune organ in your
body, which is why I want you to nurture it, along with the rest of your
digestive system. After all, without healthy digestion, you can't get the
nutrients you need for energy and good health.

WHAT YOUR POOP SAYS ABOUT YOU

As a doctor, I think beyond the dinner table. I think about what happens in our bodies after we consume all that food. And ultimately, yes, I think about what happens when our bodies are done with it. Sometimes the best way for a doctor to figure out what's going on *inside* your body is to inspect what's coming *out* of your body. Yes, I'm talking about fecal matter, excrement, or what is more commonly referred to simply as "poop." It's not a subject anyone (well, except for my gastroenterologist friends) really enjoys discussing. But the clues your poop reveals can be such valuable information in deciphering the current state of your health. So, stick with me, and read on.

Hard or pebbly: Could mean constipation or dehydration; drink more water!

Dark black: Could be sign of bleeding in upper digestive system (such as from an ulcer). Also common when eating a lot of animal proteins or taking a lot of iron supplements.

Pudding-like or watery consistency: Unformed stool may point to intolerance or sensitivity to certain foods, or a viral or bacterial infection.

Red in color: Could indicate hemorrhoids, blood from the colon caused by diverticulitis, or even cancer. However, if you're eating a lot of beets or red foods, that can also be a cause.

Soft but formed: The "A+" stool. It should, ideally, be shaped like an "S."

Pencil thin: Can indicate a narrow bowel, which is caused by a blockage or colon cancer.

Anytime you notice a change in your regular stools, schedule an appointment with your doctor right away.

How Your Digestive System Ages

If you don't want to get sick (who does?) and want to delay aging (who doesn't?), and if you want to stay in a good mood and feel wonderful in general, then a healthy digestive system should be your priority. When your digestive system is in trouble, even the most nutritious diet won't help you.

Remember the five factors of aging we discussed at the beginning of this book? Number one on that list is inflammation. Inflammation can wreak havoc on your entire body, and your digestive system is no exception. If any stop along the way on the digestive journey becomes inflamed, you can experience annoying, even painful symptoms, which can become chronic if left untreated. Long-term inflammation in the digestive tract can also wear down your stomach or intestinal lining and leave you vulnerable to a host of serious illnesses, including cancer. So, part of the game plan for protecting the health of your digestive system is to prevent or stop inflammation.

Signs of an aging digestive system include symptoms ranging from the rather benign, such as frequent constipation, to semi-serious diseases like GERD, ulcers, and irritable bowel syndrome, to the life-threatening, such as colorectal cancer. I'll discuss each one of these separately, but first I want to give you one simple solution to delay the aging of your digestive system, and that's to pop a probiotic supplement.

SUPPLEMENTS THAT SUPPORT YOUR DIGESTIVE SYSTEM

- **Probiotics:** 1–10 billion CFU (colony-forming units) or living organisms daily

  Take dosage recommended on the bottle, as products vary.

  Alternatively, eat one serving of low-fat yogurt daily.
- **Vitamin D:** 800–1,000 IU daily
- **Vitamin E:** 15 mg daily
- **Selenium:** 55 mcg daily

Why: You're reading a lot in this chapter about how probiotics can support your overall digestion and, in turn, your immunity. They can also ease digestive symptoms such as diarrhea following a round of antibiotics prescribed by your doctor. But as I mentioned earlier, you don't have to take a pill. You can also get these friendly bacteria through cultured foods such as yogurt, kefir, and acidophilus milk.

As for vitamin D, there is some early evidence that maintaining a healthy level of vitamin D in your body could reduce your risk for colorectal cancer. In China, a study of people who took supplemental vitamin E and selenium showed a lower number of deaths from stomach cancer.

The Number-One Strategy: Probiotics

Most of today's digestive distress remedies treat mainly the symptoms (providing short-term relief), and they upset the balance of bacteria in your gut. This can lead to incomplete digestion of food or to more serious disorders. If large food molecules can't pass through your intestinal wall, they'll provoke an immune response within your body, which could eventually lead to an autoimmune disorder. Faulty digestion can also prevent important nutrients from being absorbed by the body. And some scientists believe that incomplete digestion of proteins can make you more susceptible to serious disease.

Okay—probiotic supplements to the rescue. They work by crowding out bad bacteria in the gut, supporting immune function, enhancing vitamin production, and destroying toxins and carcinogens. Probiotics, when consumed properly, can work miracles, and there's little they can't do when it comes to digestive health.

When looking for a probiotic product, select a multi-strain probiotic, which means it has multiple types of friendly bacteria listed in the ingredients. You want several strains because each one has different benefits. One strain may improve overall digestion, another boosts immunity, still others ease diarrhea and digestive distress, and some promote overall colon health.

Take your probiotics on an empty stomach, and follow the manufacturer's recommendation for dosage.

Now for specific strategies that will help your digestive system function at its peak, and ultimately help you live 100 healthy years.

The Anti-Aging Essentials and Your Digestive System

#1: Movement. I don't care if this means enrolling in a hip-hop dance class, doing jumping jacks in your living room, or taking a jog around the neighborhood—movement is key for your digestion, especially in avoiding constipation.

#2: Maintain a healthy weight. Being overweight puts undue pressure on the abdominal region, and thus your digestive tract. This pressure can cause or exacerbate symptoms of GERD.

#3: Stay hydrated. Even mild dehydration can be a cause of digestive issues, especially constipation. Too little water can leave your stools dry and hard. As a result, the muscles in the lower colon and rectum will have trouble moving large dry stools from your body. This leads not only to constipation, but also to cramping, bloating, gas, hemorrhoids, bleeding, and other uncomfortable symptoms. Furthermore, drinking plenty of water can aid in diluting your stomach's acid content, thus preventing GERD.

#4: Avoid smoking. Smoking has been shown to cause harm to your stomach lining, and that makes you more vulnerable to the causes of ulcers. It also puts you at higher risk of stomach and colorectal cancers. In addition, smoking compromises the lower part of your esophagus to the point at which it can't properly get food to your stomach.

#5: Supplements. Refer to the supplement section for more information on which supplements support overall healthy digestion.

Age-Related Digestive Issues

For starters, here are the things that can go wrong with your digestive system as you get older—and what to do about them.

GERD (Gastroesophageal Reflux Disease)

This one is way too common, if you ask me. In fact, it's estimated that more than 60 million Americans feel the burn of GERD at least once a month. GERD is a chronic digestive disease that happens when stomach acid or even bile flows backward, up into your esophagus, causing heartburn. This horrible backwash of acid irritates the lining of the esophagus and causes very undesirable symptoms, such as a burning sensation in your chest, chest pain, difficulty swallowing, dry cough, or a sore throat. In essence, GERD sucks.

Supportive Strategies for GERD

- Wear clothes that fit. Clothes that are too tight or restrictive can promote this backward movement of stomach acid.

- Eat slowly, and choose smaller meals.

- Following a meal, stay on your feet or seated upright. Never lie down.

- Keep your head and neck slightly elevated while asleep. This position keeps stomach acids from moving back up in your esophagus.

Diverticulitis

After you hit age 40, you're quite likely to develop small abnormal pouches in the lining of your colon, or large intestine. If you have these, you have a condition we call diverticulosis because each pouch is called a diverticulum. About half of people over the age of 60 have diverticulosis.

In the event that those pouches become inflamed or infected, that's called diverticulitis. About 10 to 25 percent of folks who have diverticulosis (the pouches have formed in their colon) will end up with diverticulitis. This condition is often accompanied by symptoms you feel: sudden and severe abdominal pain, fever, nausea, and changing bowel habits (such as constipation or diarrhea). It's not altogether clear what causes diverticula to form in the first place, but there are some risk factors of which you should be aware: Not eating enough fiber, not getting enough exercise, and obesity can increase your chance of getting diverticulitis.

If you've been diagnosed with diverticulitis, your doctor will likely prescribe a specific diet that will often include only liquids for two days during a flare-up, in order to let your digestive system rest. After that, your physician will likely advise you to beware of certain foods such as nuts and seeds, as they can get caught in the diverticula and lead to a flare-up. Take this diagnosis very seriously, as it can lead to an intestinal perforation, which can be deadly.

Supportive Strategies for Avoiding Diverticulitis

- Make sure you consume enough fiber daily, preferably in its natural form (fruits, vegetables, and beans).
- Never ignore the urge to go "number two." If you put it off, the stool can harden and become more difficult to pass.

Irritable Bowel Syndrome (IBS)

IBS has almost become a buzzword these days, which unfortunately means that many patients self-diagnose this condition if they're experiencing abdominal pain and problems with bowel movements. But it's important that you give your physician the opportunity to rule out a lot of serious health conditions before agreeing on an IBS diagnosis. If you're experiencing abdominal pain or chronic digestive symptoms, you need to make an appointment with your doctor. These issues could be indicators of appendicitis, infections, various cancers, celiac disease, diverticulitis, an intestinal perforation, and many other serious illnesses. However, if everything else has been ruled out and your symptoms persist, IBS could be at the root of them.

Everyone experiences diarrhea, constipation, or bloating at some point in their lifetime. I can pretty much guarantee it. But when I'm describing IBS, I'm not talking about one or two bouts of watery stool following some bad shellfish (although you should watch for signs of dehydration in this case). I'm talking about a long period of time in which you have uncomfortable and irregular bowel symptoms that won't seem to stop on their own. I'm talking about that awful feeling of "will I make it to the bathroom in time?" on a very regular basis. I've had many patients get emotional when talking about the toll this condition takes on their lives.

Supportive Strategies for IBS

There are many physicians who will chalk your IBS up to stress and depression, and leave it at that. That's a traditional medical response to a poorly defined gut illness.

I don't think the problem is psychological, meaning all in your head. If that's the diagnosis you've been given, I'm afraid you'll suffer from ongoing pain and discomfort, and possibly the stigma of being diagnosed with a psychological disease.

Ask your doc to administer a simple breath test that detects the presence of intestinal bacteria. People with IBS typically show an abnormally high concentration of bacteria in their small intestines. Medically, we refer to this condition as "small intestinal bacterial overgrowth." It has been shown to be a possible cause of IBS.

If you have this overgrowth, your doctor should do two things: The first involves adding friendly bacteria to the gut in the form of probiotic supplements. The other entails selectively subtracting bad bacteria from the gut with an absorbable antibiotic, such as rifaximin (Xifaxan). Clinical studies of patients with IBS support this approach.

You can enhance this therapy with dietary recommendations. While no one specific diet works across the board to reduce IBS symptoms, I encourage these patients to experiment with adding or removing certain foods from their diet. For instance, people who consume high amounts of dairy should consider limiting lactose products for two to three weeks and see if there is any change.

Also, contrary to what you may think, fiber is extremely important here. I recommend getting increased fiber from foods, but a fiber supplement may be a solution for some—just make sure it's not loaded with sugar or artificial sweeteners. One more thing: Try limiting foods and liquids known to stimulate the digestive tract. Examples include caffeine, heavy or rich meals, and certain medications and supplements. So try this novel approach, and your bacterial overgrowth will hopefully be a thing of the past, as will your IBS.

Constipation

We all know this means being unable to have a bowel movement, but it also refers to problems during a bowel movement. Constipation is a symptom of various illnesses, but it's not an illness on its own. Traveling or going off a regular schedule can cause constipation. So can colorectal cancer, but the most common causes of constipation are a diet too low in fiber; not drinking enough water; and taking certain meds such as antidepressants or narcotics. Regular exercise is important to keep the bowels moving well, also. In people who are less active, waste doesn't move through the bowels very fast. If you go to the bathroom only three times per week, most doctors consider you to be constipated. It gets more prevalent as we get older.

Constipation is a problem of movement. If your bowels aren't "moving" properly, it could be that you aren't moving your body enough. If you're constipated, a good exercise regimen could give you great relief very quickly. Other reasons patients suffer with constipation are because they don't eat enough fiber (seeing a trend here?), the medications they take have this as a side effect, or they don't drink enough water.

DR. MIKE'S FFF'S (FAVORITE FIBER FOODS)

Fiber. It just sounds so . . . unappetizing. When I used to tell patients they needed to eat more fiber, they'd look at me as though I'd just stolen their puppy. But fiber can actually be delicious. Who doesn't enjoy biting into a juicy pear or throwing a banana in the blender for a decadent smoothie?

You may be thinking, "What? I don't have to choke down thick, gritty fiber supplement drinks while I hold my nose so I can't taste it?" That's right. I'd much prefer to see you get your fiber from the foods nature provides us anyway. Here are some of my favorite fiber foods. They're all yummy by themselves, but I included some quick recipe options you can use to dress them up, if you desire.

- One cup of raspberries (8 grams of fiber)

    Option 1: Blended with ½ cup almond milk for a raspberry shake
    Option 2: Served over one cup of oatmeal (for an extra 4 grams of fiber)
    Option 3: Sprinkled over a green garden salad
- One pear with skin (5.5 grams of fiber)

Option 1: Sliced and served with one serving sliced low-fat Swiss cheese.

Option 2: Cubed and included in a fruit salad

Option 3: Blended with lemon juice and coconut water for a pear nectar smoothie

- One cooked artichoke or one cup canned artichoke hearts (10.3 grams of fiber)

    Option 1: Steam it and dip leaves into combo of Dijon mustard, lemon juice, and seasoning.

    Option 2: Roast one can of artichoke hearts in oven, with a spritz of olive oil.

    Option 3: Include chopped artichoke hearts in pan when you bake or sauté chicken.

OTHER FFF'S

1 cup of cooked lentils (15.6 grams of fiber)

1 cup of cooked black beans (15 grams of fiber)

1 cup of lima beans (13.2 grams of fiber)

1 cup of peas (8.8 grams of fiber)

1 cup of whole-wheat spaghetti (6.2 grams of fiber)

1 cup of broccoli (5.1 grams of fiber)

¼ cup of sunflower seeds (3.9 grams of fiber)

1 banana (3.1 grams of fiber)

1 orange (3.1 grams of fiber)

1 cup of oatmeal (4 grams of fiber)

Now when I "prescribe" more fiber to patients, they rejoice. I hope you will too! And if you're wondering how much fiber to aim for each day, I go by what the National Academy of Sciences' Institute of Medicine currently recommends: Men under the age of 50 should consume about 38 grams per day and women about 25 grams. Men over the age of 50 should get 30 grams per day and women about 21 grams.

Supportive Strategies for Constipation

If you've already implemented the five anti-aging essentials in this book and you still have bathroom troubles, I think it's a good idea to look into alternative treatment options. For instance, I'm a proponent of acupuncture, as long as you choose a qualified individual who has safe practices. I also think massage can be a good option for some people because it has a relaxing effect on your muscles, hence, your bowels.

Increasing your fiber intake will also help. Fiber is key in preventing constipation. Fiber—the fragmented portions of plant foods—doesn't digest easily. Think of fiber as a train in your digestive system—along the way, nutrients, minerals, and water shuttle in and out of the train. It's essentially a vehicle for absorption along the digestive tract. Along with water and fluids, fiber adds bulk to your stools. Bulk keeps your stools moving and prevents them from being dry and hard.

Ulcers (Peptic/Stomach)

Ah, ulcers—they're perhaps one of the most colloquial and misunderstood health conditions you hear about. I'm sure we all have a parent, friend, or grandparent who has clutched his or her stomach in a moment of stress and said, "My ulcer is flaring up!" Allow me to share the truth about these little stomach sores that cause big-time pain.

First, why are they called "peptic" ulcers? Pepsin is a digestive enzyme that resides in your stomach. Depending on the location of ulcers, they have different names. For instance, a gastric ulcer is in the lining of your stomach, versus an esophageal ulcer, which is in your esophagus. Ulcer patients most commonly complain of a burning pain in their stomach region, but the pain can occur anywhere from the belly button up to the chest area.

Shockingly, between a half million and 850,000 Americans are diagnosed with peptic ulcer disease each year. And contrary to what your grandparents may say about what causes an ulcer, the truth is, it has nothing to do with spicy foods or stress. Research has now revealed that a bacterium called *Helicobacter pylori* is sometimes to blame. (Other causes include regular use of various prescription and over-the-counter medications.) However, the presence of *H. pylori* does not necessarily mean you'll get an ulcer. Conversely, there are folks who have ulcers but test negative for the bacteria. *H. Pylori* bacteria are often harmless, but sometimes they can upset the balance in your gut and ultimately cause inflammation leading to an ulcer.

So, are you asking yourself now whether the bacterium that causes ulcers is contagious? The answer is yes, it can be contagious. This strain of bacteria has been shown to spread from human to human, just like any other contagious pathogen: through food and water, kissing, and other contact.

Supportive Strategies for Ulcers

* Limit or avoid alcohol. Alcohol aggravates your stomach lining and raises the acid levels too high. If you already have an ulcer, I recommend that you don't drink alcohol at all.

* Control stress. While stress doesn't cause ulcers, it does make them worse. I know controlling your stress level is often easier said than done, but I want you to try. Regular exercise helps a lot of people manage their anxiety, as does journaling, scheduling time for relaxing and socializing, or even seeking the help of a therapist.

Hemorrhoids

There are actually two types of hemorrhoids: internal and external. When internal hemorrhoids (located inside the anal canal) swell up and get inflamed, the patient may see streaks of blood on the tissue following a bowel movement. The same symptom can occur when external hemorrhoids (located near the anal opening) get irritated.

A hemorrhoid is just a vein that has become inflamed, due to pressure. They're more common as we get older because the vessel walls weaken over time. Half of the population will experience hemorrhoids by the time they're 50 years old. Aside from the appearance of blood on the toilet paper or stool itself, other signs of hemorrhoids include a hard lump on or around the anal opening, itching, and irritation.

Supportive Strategies for Hemorrhoids

* Don't stand or sit for too long without moving around. If you work in an office, make an effort to get up and walk around a little every half hour.

- If you use bathroom time to catch up on all your reading, you may be putting yourself at increased risk for hemorrhoids.
- Try not to strain during a bowel movement. This just increases pressure down there.
- One way to avoid having to strain is to keep your stool soft and healthy by drinking plenty of fluids and eating . . . you guessed it . . . plenty of fiber.

Inflammatory Bowel Disease (IBD)

The key word in IBD is "inflammatory." Yes, it's that nasty inflammation hard at work to destroy your health yet again. If your bowels or any portion of your digestive tract are inflamed, you experience all kinds of uncomfortable and unfortunate symptoms. Patients with any IBD-related condition, such as Crohn's disease or ulcerative colitis, will experience a range of issues including abdominal pains, diarrhea, sometimes fever, rectal bleeding, loss of appetite, and unhealthy weight loss. These conditions can truly alter your life and make you feel completely miserable. Experts can't pinpoint specific causes, but there is some evidence that the digestive tract flares up in response to an attack from a virus or foreign bacteria, and that sets off a chain reaction leading to the chronic inflammation. Genetics could also be at play here; people with immediate family members who have IBD could be more likely to experience it themselves, although the science isn't completely clear at this point. If you have been diagnosed with any form of IBD, discuss with your doctor the proper nutrition and other strategies to keep the symptoms at bay.

Colorectal and Stomach Cancers

Colorectal cancer is the third most commonly diagnosed cancer in the United States and kills more than 50,000 people a year. A major risk factor for colorectal cancer is age, with more than 90 percent of cases occurring in people 50 years and older.

Possible signs of this cancer include:

- A change in bowel habits
- Blood (either bright red or very dark) in the stool
- Diarrhea, constipation, or feeling that the bowel does not empty completely
- Stools that are narrower than usual
- Frequent gas pains, bloating, fullness, or cramps
- Weight loss for no known reason
- Feeling very tired
- Vomiting

Polyps can form in the stomach lining where there's inflammation. When these polyps become malignant (cancerous), they're called adeno-carcinomas.

Supportive Strategies for Preventing Colorectal and Stomach Cancers

- Eat less sodium. Research has linked too much salt in the diet to a higher risk for a stomach cancer diagnosis. Look, there's enough sodium in our food as it is. Throw away your salt shaker and avoid packaged and processed foods, which are known to be high in sodium. Try using garlic as a seasoning instead, since there is an association between increased garlic intake and reduced risk of some cancers, including stomach cancer.

- Eat more fruits and veggies, especially the ones high in vitamin C and beta carotene. There's promising research that diets rich in yellow, orange, and dark green veggies and fruits can put you in a lower-risk category for stomach cancer.

Before you begin Cycle 2: Rebuild, take this quiz to find out the state of your current digestive health. Then, after you complete the 17 Day Plan, take this quiz again to see how much you improved your score!

Is Your Digestive System on Its Way to 100 Happy, Healthy Years?

1. **How often do you have a full or bloated feeling in your stomach, especially after eating?**

    A. Daily ☐ 0 points
    B. Often ☐ 1 point
    C. Infrequently ☐ 3 points
    D. Never ☐ 4 points

2. **How often do you have loose stools (diarrhea)?**

    A. Daily ☐ 0 points
    B. Often ☐ 1 point
    C. Infrequently ☐ 3 points
    D. Never ☐ 4 points

3. **How often do you suffer constipation?**

    A. Daily ☐ 0 points
    B. Often ☐ 1 point
    C. Infrequently ☐ 2 points
    D. Never ☐ 4 points

4. **Do you avoid eating certain foods because they make you feel uncomfortable?**

    A. Yes ☐ 0 points　　　　B. No ☐ 4 points

5. **How often do you experience abdominal cramps or pains?**

    A. Daily ☐ 0 points
    B. Often ☐ 1 point
    C. Infrequently ☐ 3 points
    D. Never ☐ 4 points

6. **Have you ever taken an antibiotic for more than one month at a time?**

    A. Yes ☐ 0 points　　　B. No ☐ 4 points

7. **How often do you have bowel movements?**

    A. Less than twice a week □ 0 points
    B. Less than three times a week □ 1 point
    C. Four to five times a week □ 3 points
    D. Every day □ 4 points

8. **What color is your poop most of the time?**

    A. Yellowish to greenish □ 0 points
    B. Light brown □ 3 points
    C. Dark brown □ 4 points

9. **Have you ever experienced black stools?**

    A. Yes □ 0 points   B. No □ 4 points

10. **Have you ever experienced blood in your stool?**

    A. Yes □ 0 points   B. No □ 4 points

11. **Do your bowel movements have an unusually terrible odor?**

    A. Yes □ 0 points   B. Not really □ 4 points

12. **How often do you have cravings for sweets or starches?**

    A. Daily □ 0 points
    B. Several times a week □ 1 point
    C. A few times a week □ 2 points
    D. Rarely □ 4 points

13. **How often do you experience indigestion?**

    A. Daily □ 0 points
    B. Several times a week □ 1 point
    C. A few times a week □ 2 points
    D. Never □ 4 points

14. **How often do you experience belching or flatulence?**

    A. Daily □ 0 points
    B. Several times a week □ 1 point
    C. A few times a week □ 2 points
    D. Never □ 4 points

Scoring:

0–11: URGENT; see your doctor ASAP about your digestive health.

12–22: DANGEROUS; change your risky digestive system routines
immediately.

23–33: MODERATELY RISKY; start incorporating more of my
suggested changes into your life to improve your digestion.

34–44: AVERAGE; you have room for additional change.

45–56: EXCELLENT; stay on this positive course.

Your gut needs a delicate balance of nutrients to do its best work for you, so listen to its needs and do everything in your power to meet them. Symptoms having to do with digestion are often uncomfortable and embarrassing, and they can severely alter your mood and overall quality of life. The steps to take in order to avoid these problems really aren't that hard, when you think about it. I hope you have a little more respect for the journey of digestion, and that you're ready to do your part to support it in order to experience 100 years of digestive health.

CHAPTER 9

Feeling Hormonal?

A s we inch toward middle age and beyond, some of us are desperate to find the proverbial Fountain of Youth. Many longevity experts believe that magic elixir is found in hormones. Part of the endocrine system, hormones are chemicals that act like messengers. They're manufactured in one part of the body, usually a gland, and travel to other parts to help regulate how cells and organs do their jobs. A good example is the hormone insulin. It's made in the pancreas but released into the bloodstream to help control levels of glucose (blood sugar) in the body.

Can proper hormonal balance slow the hands of time? I agree with some experts that hormones play an important role as we age. But when people take it too far and start abusing things like human growth hormone (HGH) or improperly using hormone replacement therapies (HRTs), that's where we can run into trouble. My position is this: Taking sex hormones like estrogen or testosterone, human growth hormone (HGH), or DHEA (a building block of sex hormones) is not a stand-alone anti-aging intervention—although these hormones show promising benefits for anti-aging when used with other measures, such as those I've discussed so far and others I'm about to explain.

Endocrine System 101

Endo means "inside" in Greek, and *crinis* means "secrete." Thus, your endocrine system's primary function is to produce and secrete hormones inside certain glands. The glands I'm referring to are your hypothalamus, pancreas, adrenals, ovaries and testicles, pituitary, thyroid, pineal, thymus, and parathyroid. The hormones produced in these glands have many different jobs, ranging from controlling the use of glucose (sugar) in your body to maintaining your metabolism and keeping your immune system strong, even creating reproductive cells. Yes, there's a lot going on with your endocrine system! Here's a more detailed look inside:

Thyroid and parathyroid. Your thyroid is located at the front of your neck, and its shape is reminiscent of a bow tie. It primarily produces thyroxine (T-4) and triiodothyronine (T-3). The parathyroid glands are four smaller glands attached to the thyroid. Among other things, the hormones produced by your thyroid control your metabolism, while PTH (parathyroid hormone) properly regulates the use of calcium in building your bones.

Pituitary gland. This pea-sized gland is inside your brain (although it's not actually part of your brain) and it acts like the "captain" to all your other endocrine glands, sending messages that encourage them to produce their own hormones. Along with other hormones, the pituitary gland secretes human growth hormone.

Hypothalamus. This is actually part of your brain, and it creates something called neurohormones. The endocrine and nervous systems work closely together, and this organ is a perfect example of their connectivity or entwinement. The hormones made here have an effect on the pituitary gland as well as on others. It plays a huge part in regulating your temperature, blood pressure, sleep habits, sexual activity, moods, and many other bodily functions.

Ovaries. These female reproductive glands, about the size of an almond, produce reproductive cells and sex hormones responsible for giving women their distinctly female attributes. Ovaries produce primarily estrogen and progesterone, but they also produce small amounts of testosterone.

Testes. These male reproductive organs, generally the size of a large grape and located below the penis inside the scrotum, are in charge of creating sperm (the male reproductive cells) and testosterone.

Pancreas. This gland sits behind the stomach and creates insulin, which is a vital component in your body's ability to properly utilize glucose. Having a healthy pancreas is necessary for healthy digestion.

Adrenals. These are two glands situated right above your kidneys. They produce multiple hormones, specifically in response to stress. The function of the hormones produced here has to do with fight or flight, metabolism, blood sugar levels, and more.

Pineal gland. The pineal gland is close to the center of your brain. It makes melatonin, which regulates your sleep patterns.

How Your Endocrine System Ages

Ideally, your body synthesizes just the right amount of the many different hormones needed to keep you healthy, but as you age, this synthesis changes. Essentially, production slows. The hormone assembly line doesn't move at the same pace that it did in your 20s. What does this mean for your health? One effect is a decreased ability to respond to various types of stresses due to a reduction in hypothalamic hormones. Another physical response is less muscle mass, caused by a decrease in human growth hormone.

The adrenal glands create a hormone called aldosterone, which helps maintain your hydration levels. Because you make less of this hormone as you age, you run a higher risk of dehydration. (This is just another great reason to always drink plenty of water!)

Also, over time, your thyroid may start to develop nodules. This may be something your general practitioner can actually feel during a routine check. An aging thyroid and decreased production in thyroid hormones play a role in a decreased metabolism. Metabolism is your body's food-to-fuel process. It helps turn protein, carbs, and fats into energy. The more efficient your metabolism, the better your body can burn fat. Actually, your metabolism hits a peak when you're around 20 years old and it starts to slow slightly at that point. That's why it gets harder to keep a slim figure as we age. Fortunately, you can charge up your metabolism with regular exercise (particularly weight training) and a prudent diet of natural foods and lean protein.

The pancreas also experiences changes as it ages. You may produce less insulin over time, and the insulin you do produce may become less effective. Remember, the role of insulin is to allow the sugar you consume to become energy you burn. So the decreased production can lead to changes in how your body reacts to sugar in the foods you eat. The best tactic for preventing insulin problems is to manage your portion sizes and sugar consumption. I advise my patients to do that the easy way: Use your hands. A fist represents the amount of veggies and fruit to eat at meals; the palm of your hand equals a reasonable quantity of protein, such as chicken, fish, or lean meat. A cupped hand represents a serving of pasta, rice, or whole-grain cereal, and the size of your thumb equals the amount of oil, salad dressing, nut butter, mayonnaise, or other fat you should eat.

The pituitary gland has actually been shown to shrink in size as we grow older. As you can imagine, the smaller size does lower its effectiveness. Since the pituitary gland is in charge of many other endocrine functions, a malfunction in the pituitary can show up in symptoms attributed to the thyroid, sexual organs, and adrenals. Pituitary disorders can cause decreased libido, headaches, irregular periods, fertility problems, and a host of other issues.

In short, because the structures within the endocrine system are comingled with each other, as well as with your other body systems, you really want to preserve the health and vitality of this system. Here's how!

SUPPLEMENTS THAT SUPPORT YOUR ENDOCRINE SYSTEM

- **Calcium:** 1,000 mg total daily
- **Vitamin D:** 800–1,000 IU total daily
- **Green tea:** one cup total daily

Why: Hyperthyroidism, in particular, can quicken the aging of your bones and even cause them to get thinner, so supplementing with calcium and vitamin D is an especially good idea if you have this disorder. But did you know that soda and other caffeinated products can actually cause you to absorb less of the calcium you're consuming? Table salt can also leach calcium from your bones, increasing your risk of osteoporosis. So, even if you're taking the recommended amounts of calcium every day, you might be undoing the good you've done if you're washing it down with cola and sprinkling salt on all your meals.

Green tea—either caffeinated or decaf—packs an antioxidant punch that can keep you healthy and could even give your metabolism a boost. You can get it either caffeinated or decaffeinated. But don't ruin its benefits by adding sugar.

The Number-One Strategy: Manage Stress

The top priority of the endocrine system is to maintain something called homeostasis within your body. It wants you and your health to be consistently stable. Sounds good, right? Who doesn't like stability? So, what stands between you and homeostasis? One word: stress. And since a certain amount of stress in life is inevitable, your endocrine system has a built-in plan for protecting you from it. The glands of your endocrine system release certain hormones in response to whatever type of stress is jeopardizing your health. Now, stress comes in many forms. Perhaps it's bad financial news or a family dispute; maybe it's a minor car accident or even just a cold. Whatever the cause, stress sets your endocrine system into action to get you back to homeostasis.

However, when stress goes on for an extended period, your endocrine system has to work overtime to produce the correct amount of hormones to keep all your bodily systems functioning properly. This overtime can lead to problems with the cardiovascular system, including high blood pressure. It can also cause decreased immunity. Did you ever notice how you're more likely to catch a cold or the flu when you're stressed out? It can even have a negative effect on the reproductive system, leading to changes in women's menstruation and men's testosterone and sperm production. Yes, a hormonal imbalance due to long-term stress can have serious effects on the entire body.

Stress is insidious. So many patients I see are walking around at maximum stress levels, and the scariest part is that they don't even realize it. Stress has almost become a way of life for them. In my opinion, long-term stress is a choice. No, you never choose for bad things to happen, and that's not what I mean. But the way you react to potentially stressful situations is fully within your control. I truly believe that if you can learn the keys to managing stress in your life, you can avoid many health problems along the way and greatly increase your chances of living 100 happy, healthy years.

Stress Reduction Strategies

Learning to take control of your stress levels and understanding that *you* decide, to some extent at least, how much stress you're allowing your body to feel is a key element in boosting the health of your endocrine system, as well as your entire body. You may think that de-stressing can be accomplished only at an expensive spa, on an extravagant vacation, or with the help of a pricey therapist. Those things can be great, but they're not essential to managing your stress on a daily basis. I promise!

Rate your stress. First, know your stress level. Ask yourself throughout the day where you are on a scale of one to 10 for stress. One is calm, relaxed, but alert; 10 is when sirens are blaring in your head, your palms are sweating, and you're feeling major, massive stress. If you rate your stress level within the range of six to 10 a lot of the time, it's time for some serious changes.

Make a stress solution list. Make a two-column list, with everything that is stressing you out in the left column. Just the act of writing all these things down on paper can be helpful; it somehow takes their power away. When you have the whole stress list done, start on the right column, which is a list of possible solutions. Even if the first thing that comes to mind is outrageous (e.g., "quit job and run away to Bora Bora"), write it down! Don't expect yourself to come up with a realistic solution for every single stressor right off the bat, but keep this list close and when you think of something, add it. Soon, you'll discover that every little detail causing you stress can be managed, worked out, delegated, or deleted.

Perceive "movement" differently. Movement has a special effect on psychological stress; when you exercise, your brain becomes occupied with maintaining all your functions while you physically exert yourself. It's focusing on getting oxygen to your heart and muscles and keeping everything moving safely and effectively. That means it's less preoccupied with dwelling on all of life's stressors. Your head feels "clear." (All that fresh oxygen sure helps, too!) But, for many of you, daily exercise might end up on your list of things stressing you out! If the thought of dragging yourself to the gym and plodding along on the treadmill absolutely turns your stomach, let's make an effort to change your perception.

Exercise can be fun. It's true! It should be something you look forward to because it's sort of an escape from the daily grind. Ask yourself to remember the last time you had fun while you were breathing hard and sweating. Was it when you were dancing with your partner or a group of friends years ago? Then get yourself a workout DVD filled with fun and fast-paced dance moves and throw a dance party in your living room! If it was when you were playing kickball in fifth grade, then join an adult kickball league (yes, they exist!). If it was when you were jumping on the bed as a kid, get yourself a small trampoline or rebounder, play some fun music, and laugh your head off while jumping up and down! Seriously, folks, there's no reason you have to dread exercise. With all the benefits it has to offer, I strongly encourage you to find a way to enjoy 30 minutes of daily movement. Get creative!

Use your time tools. Many people who are stressed out, strung out, frazzled, and overwhelmed also happen to be people who don't have great time management skills. No matter how many daily tasks you're juggling, there's always a way to manage your time efficiently so you're not constantly running late and feeling drained. You probably have email, which means you probably have access to some type of calendar that will give you reminders. That's a great tool you can use to keep a detailed schedule. If syncing your and your family's agenda is a problem, find a common area in the home (possibly the kitchen) to create a master calendar. Make sure everyone writes on it so you're all on the same page. Bottom line: Find a way to better organize your time. It will help you feel more in control and less anxious.

Know when you need help. Anxiety disorders are very real and can be devastating. If you suspect that you have a psychological problem, seek the advice of a counselor or therapist. Find someone you trust. Help is available; it may be that you'll benefit from cognitive behavioral therapy, counseling, or possibly medication.

The Anti-Aging Essentials and Your Endocrine System

#1: Movement. Especially if you're stressed, you want to exercise to maintain the health of your endocrine system because it can slow down the release of stress-related hormones. Remember those NEAT (nonexercise activity thermogenesis) movements that you should do throughout the day! Or find ways to "sneak" exercise in, such as by doing lunges while you vacuum or calf raises while you're waiting in line at the grocery store. Sometimes it can feel great to release stress by enrolling in a kickboxing class, or hitting a punching bag.

#2: Maintain a healthy weight. If you're obese, that extra weight can trigger something we call metabolic syndrome, which is a combination of risk factors for type 2 diabetes, heart disease, and stroke. Visceral fat, the kind that lives under your abdominal wall and chokes the life out of your organs, is especially dangerous in relation to your risk for diabetes. According to the researchers at the Harvard School of Public Health, when it comes to type 2 diabetes, the top factor in determining whether someone will develop the disease is if the person is overweight or obese. Part of the reason why being overweight increases your odds of a diabetes diagnosis has to do with how your cells process sugar, which can lead to high blood sugar. It can also cause the insulin-producing cells to have to work even harder to keep blood sugar normalized, which can ultimately lead to cellular failure. Thus, being overweight or obese negatively impacts your whole body, even down to the tiniest cells.

#3: Stay hydrated. Maintaining proper hydration every day can actually help your metabolism. One study at the University of Utah found that adults who drank eight to twelve 8-ounce glasses of water per day burned more calories than people who were dehydrated. Burning extra calories just by drinking water? That sure sounds good to me!

#4: Avoid smoking. Smoking can interfere with the functioning of your endocrine system, specifically the thyroid. It increases the risk of Graves' disease (a form of hyperthyroidism) and type 2 diabetes.

#5: Supplements. Refer to my list of supplements that specifically support your endocrine system.

Age-Related Endocrine Issues

First, let's take a tour of a few of the things that can go wrong with your endocrine system as you age, and of course, how to prevent them or at least slow them down.

Type 2 Diabetes

The American Diabetes Association reports that over 25 million Americans are living with diabetes, 90 to 95 percent of whom have type 2 diabetes. The disease of diabetes boils down to an issue of the hormone insulin. It means that the pancreas either doesn't produce enough insulin to manage glucose (sugar) in the blood or the body just isn't using it properly. I'm going to spend a bit more time on this topic, not because I want to scare you, but because I want you to be informed. Did you know that the Centers for Disease Control estimate that, if we continue down the path we're on, one in three adults in America could be diagnosed with diabetes by the year 2050? That's a horrifying statistic—and it doesn't have to be that way. The CDC also reports that diabetes is the seventh-leading cause of death in the United States. Furthermore, people with diabetes are at least twice as likely to develop heart disease or have a stroke as others. It's also the number-one cause of new cases of blindness in people 20 to 74 years old. You're at higher risk for diabetes if:

- You're over the age of 45
- You're carrying extra weight around the waist (and maybe other places too)
- Your HDL is under 35 mg/dL
- You have high blood pressure
- You don't move your body enough!
- Someone else in your family has or had diabetes

I'm not saying you're doomed to a diabetes diagnosis if you meet one or more of these criteria. But I do want you to make it your top priority to lower the risk factors you can control.

Supportive Strategies for Preventing Type 2 Diabetes

Get screened. If you have risk factors, it's a good idea to get tested. Knowledge is power! Your doctor may perform a fasting blood sugar test or glycated hemoglobin (A1C) test; they can be helpful in diagnosis and prevention.

Choose foods wisely. Eating a healthy diet is simpler than you think. The first step is to become conscious of what you're eating. Start by making an effort to eat 14 grams of fiber for every 1,000 calories you eat. Why do I mention fiber specifically? It seems to have a positive effect on your blood sugar levels.

Switch up your oils. Try using coconut oil in your cooking occasionally. Coconut oil is composed of medium-chain fatty acids, which produce energy, rather than the long-chain fatty acids found in animal fats like lard and butter. Using a combination of different types of fats has been linked to a reduction in type 2 diabetes risk as well as heart disease. So, it's healthier to switch between your oils so you're not consistently cooking with the same type.

Thyroid Issues

There are three conditions I'll emphasize here. The first is hypothyroidism, which refers to an underactive thyroid—one that doesn't produce enough of certain hormones needed to maintain your metabolism and various chemical reactions in your body. The American Association of Clinical Endocrinologists estimates that 27 million American adults have an underactive or overactive thyroid. Women have about a seven times higher risk than men for issues with the thyroid, specifically hypothyroidism, as they get older. Common symptoms of hypothyroidism are unexplained fatigue, constipation, hoarseness, puffy and pale face, inexplicable weight gain, and a general feeling of sluggishness.

The second issue is hyperthyroidism, which is when your thyroid is overactive and produces too much thyroxine, a vital hormone in your metabolism. Typical signs are sudden weight loss, fast heartbeat, excess sweating or a feeling of nervousness, bigger appetite than normal, heat sensitivity, and frequent bowel movements. It's also possible to have no signs at all! This is another reason why thyroid testing is imperative.

Finally, there is thyroid cancer. Cancer of any type sounds very scary. But there's some good news about thyroid cancer. If you're diagnosed with stage I or II of the various types of thyroid cancer, your survival rate is nearly 100 percent. That said, you still want to be diligent about your thyroid health and looking for symptoms of thyroid cancer. People who have had a goiter, or have family members with a goiter, are at a higher risk of thyroid cancer, as are people with certain genetic syndromes or who have been exposed to radiation. If you feel a lump in your neck area, pain that doesn't go away after a couple of days, or trouble swallowing, speak to your doctor about some thyroid testing.

Supportive Strategies for a Healthy Thyroid

Have your thyroid checked. The recommendation from the American Thyroid Association is for people over age 35 to get their thyroid tested every five years. You can also perform a self-exam. It's a good idea to perform this test twice a year to look for any changes in your thyroid. Simply look in the mirror at your neck, lean your head back slightly, and then swallow. Your thyroid is around the center of your neck and it protrudes slightly; you'll see it move when you swallow. Do this a few times, looking for anything abnormal on or near your thyroid.

Watch for symptoms. Especially if you're female, you should be on the lookout for subtle changes in your health. Don't take it to the level of paranoia, but I don't want you to brush it off if you've noticed a feeling of lethargy, sudden weight gain, or other symptoms of hypothyroidism. There are medications that can control this, so give your doctor a chance to help you!

Get plenty of calcium and vitamin D. Hyperthyroidism, in particular, can quicken the aging of your bones and even cause them to get thinner, so supplementing with calcium and vitamin D is a good idea.

Consume enough iodine. Since our salt was iodized back in the 1970s, we doctors haven't seen as many patients who are severely lacking in iodine.

However, the more conscious people become about their sodium intake, the more we're on the lookout for the effects of low iodine. Foods to incorporate in your diet are shellfish or fish, eggs, onions, radishes, parsley, and kelp.

Snackin' on Seaweed

If you've recently walked down the aisles of a health food store, or even some mainstream grocery stores, you may have noticed a couple of rows of pre-packaged seaweed treats. If you aren't the adventurous type, you may have passed right by the strange-looking snacks on your way to the spaghetti sauce aisle. But let me try to convince you to give them a try, or better yet, make them on your own! I mostly recommend trying roasted seaweed; it's a low-calorie yet filling snack that can act as a healthy replacement to potato chips because it has a nice little crunch.

Seaweed also happens to contain some healthy vitamins and minerals including potassium, vitamin K, calcium, vitamin C, magnesium, and iodine. While it's important to get iodine in your diet, I don't really see many patients with an iodine deficiency. That's mostly because of the amount of iodized salt we consume in our typical American diet. On the other hand, as more and more people have to carefully monitor their salt intake, we may start seeing more patients experience negative effects on their thyroid from too little iodine. An iodine-deficient diet can cause goiters, or enlarged thyroid.

Here's my prescription: especially if you're restricting salt, give roasted seaweed snacks a try. Here's how to make them on your own!

4 large sheets of toasted nori (found in the Asian aisle of your grocery store)
1 teaspoon sesame oil

Preheat the oven to 275 degrees F. Using a knife or kitchen shears, cut the sheets of toasted nori into squares, about the size of potato chips. Brush a light coating of sesame oil on both sides of the squares. Bake them for 10 to 15 minutes, until they are crispy. Serve as a snack!

Serving size: 10 to 12 bite-size crisps

Slower Metabolism

Metabolism is how your body changes the nutrients in the food and drink you consume into energy. And energy is something you need, literally, all the time. It's not only necessary for when you're going on a jog or doing work in the yard. Energy is essential for your body to function on every level.

As you get older, your metabolism slows down. So, you want to do everything you can to fuel its fires and keep it going strong. The faster your metabolism is, the more energy you have and the better your body can process nutrients.

Supportive Strategies to Speed Up Metabolism

Eat breakfast. Your mom always told you that breakfast is the most important meal of the day. She was right . . . again! I recommend eating within 30 minutes of waking up, to jolt your metabolism out of its "rest" mode and into "burn" mode. If you skip it, you're basically asking your body to store calories as fat because it's preparing for the worst-case scenario: no food! Plus, it's just common sense that you're more likely to overdo it at your next meal if you let yourself go hungry for too long.

Strike a balance with lean protein. You tend to burn more calories during the digestion of proteins. One study found that the "sweet spot" amount of lean protein (think: chicken breasts, lean turkey, lean beef, tofu, etc.) is one-third of your total daily calories. So if you're eating 2,000 calories per day, about 650 calories should come from lean protein products.

Maintain a sleep routine. If you don't get enough sleep on a regular basis, your metabolism won't function at its best. Also, have you ever noticed how much hungrier you feel after a restless night? The research isn't clear yet, but it's possible that lack of sleep wreaks havoc on appetite-regulating hormones. Try to get the same amount of sleep every night—don't leave all your sleeping to the weekends!

Drink ice water. In some people, drinking ice cold water may boost your metabolism. The reason: Your body goes into a bit of overdrive to heat up its core temperature. The effects aren't proven to be long-term, but we'll take what we can get!

Work out late in the day. If you can manage an evening workout without it disrupting your sleep, I say try it. There's some evidence that it could keep your metabolism from dropping as low at night, which means you're burning more calories even as you get your shut-eye. But if the PM workouts make you hungry and cause you to snack late at night, be careful to choose higher protein foods and stay away from the carbs.

WARNING: HGH ANTI-AGING FAD

You may have recently heard of people turning to HGH injections in an effort to turn back the hands of time. You'll hear claims of this "miracle" drug increasing libido, giving a youthful glow to skin, even eradicating gray hair! But the fact is, HGH replacement is safe only for people who actually have a growth hormone deficiency, which is quite rare. It's not a miracle or a fountain of youth, and it's not FDA-approved for anti-aging uses. HGH injection can cause side effects including joint and muscle pain, swelling, and enlargement of breast tissue in men. It could even contribute to risk factors for diabetes, heart disease, and cancer. Because there have been limited studies conducted on it, we don't actually know all the risks it carries. And that's enough for me to say that HGH injections, unless prescribed to you by a legitimate doctor for a legitimate and approved cause, should be avoided.

Now take this quiz to find out how healthy your endocrine system is. Then, after you complete Cycle 2: Rebuild, take this quiz again to see how much you improved your score!

Is Your Endocrine System on Its Way to 100 Happy, Healthy Years?

1. **In the past week, have about one-third of your daily calories come from lean protein?**

    A. Yes ☐ 4 points   B. No ☐ 0 points

2. **Have you recently experienced unexplained weight gain or weight loss?**

    A. Yes ☐ 0 points   B. No ☐ 4 points

3. **Are you of normal body weight for your height?**

    A. Normal (within a few pounds) ☐ 4 points
    B. Need to lose five to 10 pounds ☐ 2 points
    C. More than 15 pounds overweight ☐ 0 points

4. **If you're over the age of 45, have you ever had your thyroid checked?**

    A. Yes ☐ 4 points   B. No ☐ 0 points

5. **Does anyone in your immediate family have diabetes?**

    A. Yes ☐ 0 points   B. No ☐ 4 points

6. **How many times did you do cardio exercise in the last week?**

    A. One time or not at all ☐ 0 points
    B. Two or three times ☐ 2 points
    C. Four times or more ☐ 4 points

7. **Do you have difficulty sleeping?**

    A. Yes ☐ 0 points   B. No ☐ 4 points

8. **Do you feel sluggish or tired?**

    A. Yes ☐ 0 points   B. No ☐ 4 points

9. **Does your energy drop in the afternoon?**

   A. Yes, very often ☐ 0 points
   B. Sometimes ☐ 2 points
   C. Never ☐ 4 points

10. **Have you had any change in bowel movements?**

   A. Yes ☐ 0 points   B. No ☐ 4 points

11. **Are you stressed?**

   A. Yes, all the time! ☐ 0 points
   B. Occasionally (not every day) ☐ 3 points
   C. No, I'm cool as a cucumber. ☐ 4 points

12. **How many times do you eat per day?**

   A. One large meal and snacks ☐ 1 point
   B. Three large meals ☐ 2 points
   C. Four to six small meals throughout day ☐ 4 points

13. **Have you ever developed diabetes during pregnancy?**

   A. Yes ☐ 0 points   B. No ☐ 4 points

14. **Do you eat 25 grams of fiber per day if you're a woman and 38 grams per day if you're a man?**

   A. Yes ☐ 4 points   B. No ☐ 0 points

Scoring:

0–11: URGENT; if you're experiencing unexplained weight gain, extreme lethargy, or other alarming symptoms, see your doctor or endocrinologist for an evaluation.

12–22: DANGEROUS; stop your bad habits and start some good ones immediately to improve the functioning of your endocrine system. If any symptoms don't improve, see your doctor.

23–33: MODERATELY RISKY; start doing more of my recommendations for a healthy endocrine system.

34–44: AVERAGE; you have room for additional change.

45–56: EXCELLENT; stay on this positive course.

I understand that reducing your stress could seem like an insurmountable task and that preventing diabetes if you have a family history may seem like an uphill battle. But I promise that both are possible. So now that you understand how your endocrine system works and how it regulates your body's functions, I urge you to take care of it because if you do, you will have boundless energy and avoid many life-shortening diseases. Simple changes in your daily living can work wonders for your endocrine system and on helping you look, feel, and act younger than ever!

CHAPTER 10

Make No Bones About It

As we get older, our muscles begin to weaken. Everyday tasks, such as walking up a flight of stairs, carrying suitcases, or lugging groceries, become more difficult. We can feel unbalanced on our feet and tire easily.

There is also the risk of falling and getting hurt. I'm talking about all the ways we can injure ourselves, including bruises, fractures, cuts, and contusions—there are hundreds of different bad things that can happen to the human body when it endures a fall.

And speaking of falls, one in three people age 65 or older will suffer a fall. And worse than that, it appears that your odds of dying from injuries related to a fall have risen quite a bit over the past 10 years. This is sad news, and it keeps us doctors busy.

I would rather that *you* be the busy one, getting out of the house and doing things you love to do no matter what your age—play sports, go shopping, ski, attend a political convention, or whatever it may be, without worrying about whether you'll fall and break something. You can have a great life by taking care of your musculoskeletal system—your muscles, bones, and joints. Without these vital body parts, we wouldn't be able to stand, walk, or even sit, so taking care of them is essential, starting right now.

Musculoskeletal System 101

Muscles

Your body has more than 650 muscles, which make up half of your body weight. Muscles are attached to bones by tough tissues called tendons. They help your muscles move your bones.

We have three different kinds of muscle: skeletal, smooth, and cardiac.

138

Skeletal muscle is the kind you work when you go to the gym. It is found throughout your body, mostly in the legs, arms, abs, chest, neck, and face. Skeletal muscles are called "striated" because they are composed of fibers that have horizontal stripes that you can see under a microscope. These muscles hold your skeleton together, give your body shape, and help it with everyday movements.

Other muscles in the body are "smooth" muscles. They are made up of fibers but are not striated. These aren't the typical muscles you see on a bodybuilder. The smooth muscles are inside your body, even inside your organs, including the ones lining your stomach, small intestine, and colon. You can't decide when you're going to "flex" these muscles; your brain actually sends a signal to them when they're needed to go into action. These muscles help break up food, move it through the digestive system, and also squeeze blood through the walls of blood vessels to help maintain blood pressure.

The third type of muscle found in your body is cardiac muscle. Every time you feel your heart beat in your chest, just imagine all those cardiac muscle fibers at work to pump blood throughout your body.

Bones

Your body has 206 bones, which begin to develop before you are born. Throughout the rest of your life, there is a magical "remodeling" process going on in your bones. Think *Extreme Makeover: Bone Edition*. Essentially, your skeleton continues to redesign and even transform on the cellular level. You have three types of bone cells: osteocytes, osteoclasts, and osteoblasts. Think of them as all playing roles on a construction site. First are the osteocytes, which act sort of like cranes. They're responsible for picking up and moving materials (nutrients and waste) from one place to another. Next, the osteoclasts: I compare them to the wrecking ball or bulldozer. They dismantle bone in order for it to be rebuilt stronger. Lastly, the osteoblasts: They're like the actual construction workers who are building the new bone material. They also repair damaged areas in your bone.

Embedded in the protein fibers of bones are needle-like crystals of calcium, phosphorus, and other strengthening material. You always hear about the importance of calcium for bone health, right? Rightly so! Calcium provides the structural strength that lets bones support your weight and anchor your muscles. Calcium that is not used right away is stored in your bones. The level of certain vitamins and minerals you take in, especially vitamin D and calcium, directly affects how much calcium is stored.

And there's even more magic that occurs within your bones. Inside many bones is your bone marrow, where most of your blood cells are made. The bone marrow is filled with stem cells, which produce red blood cells and platelets, and some types of white blood cells. Red blood cells transport oxygen to the body's tissues, and platelets regulate blood clotting when you cut yourself. White blood cells help your body fight infection.

Bones are attached to other bones by long, fibrous straps called ligaments. Cartilage, a flexible, rubbery substance in the joints, protects bones where they rub against each other, such as in your knees and elbows.

Joints

Joint pain is one of the most common complaints as we get older, so I'm guessing you can easily think of a few examples of joints. Your knees, hips, and elbows are all examples of where two (or more) bones meet. You know the old song: The thigh bone's connected to the hip bone . . . and so on. Joints give you flexibility—how would you even walk if you couldn't bend your knees?

When joints get creaky and stiff, that means trouble, as in arthritis or something else that restricts movement. These are ailments that make quality of life pretty miserable, so we want to avoid them as long as we can. (Or better yet, forever!)

How the Musculoskeletal System Ages

The aging of your musculoskeletal system is what can really make you feel old. Bones are strong, but obviously they can break or weaken. Muscles can also weaken, and joints (tendons, ligaments, and cartilage) can be damaged by injury or disease. There are plenty of problems that can affect the bones, muscles, and joints as we age. Here are a few:

Skeletal decline. Between the ages of 30 and 40 you start gradually losing bone mass. Bones get thinner and relatively weaker from there. The number of osteoblasts (bone-building cells) begins to drop, while the number of osteoclasts (cells that break down bone) remains the same. What happens is that osteoclasts remove calcium faster than osteoblasts can regrow it, so your bones weaken. Weak bones mean increased likelihood of breaks.

Male/female hormone issues. You might not realize it, but hormones—vital chemical messengers in the body—are related to bone health and bone loss. Three main hormones are involved in the complex process of bone formation. One is parathyroid hormone, produced by small glands in your neck. Parathyroid hormone releases calcium from the bone; as you get older, this hormone increases in the body. This means that the rate at which calcium exits bone is greater than the rate at which calcium is absorbed into bone.

Testosterone and estrogen are also both involved in bone maintenance. Testosterone stimulates bone formation, and estrogen protects against bone loss. As you get older, there is a natural decline in these hormones—a process that also contributes to the loss of bone. Guys, you lose testosterone, and this affects your bone mass, albeit very slowly. Ladies, after menopause, there's a dramatic decrease in estrogen, leading to a potentially rapid loss of bone. The incidence of bone fractures is two to three times higher in women than in men.

Size and power of muscles. With age, your muscles lose some size and power, as skeletal muscle fibers become smaller in diameter. The net effect is less muscular strength, reduced endurance, and a tendency to tire rapidly. And remember the heart is a muscle too, and its performance can decline as well.

Loss of muscle mass accelerates around age 75. This can make you frail and increases your risk of falls and fractures. Your muscles feel weaker, and you'll tire more easily. Although exercise is the best remedy, you may not feel like being active, which in turn further jeopardizes your muscle mass. It can be an ugly cycle if you let it go too far.

Bone malfunctions. Osteoporosis, which leaves bone tissue brittle and thin, is the most common type of bone disease. It causes bones to break more easily, and the spine sometimes begins to weaken. Researchers estimate that one out of five American women over the age of 50 has osteoporosis. About half of all women over the age of 50 will suffer a fracture of the hip, wrist, or vertebra (bones of the spine).

Osteoarthritis (OA). It's happened to a lot of us: Spend too much time running, attending high-impact aerobic dance classes, or skiing, and you'll ache afterward. Maybe your knee joint swells or there's some redness. You pop a couple of pain relievers and feel fine . . . but you're left thinking, "Hey, I'm no spring chicken anymore!"

For others, the pain keeps on keeping on, sometimes for years—and it's not a case of sore or overworked muscles. It's osteoarthritis, the most common joint disorder we doctors see, one that is painful to witness because our patients really suffer. It is caused by aging and wear and tear on joints—in other words, joint injury. When the cartilage around joints breaks down and wears away, the bones rub together. This causes pain, swelling, and stiffness. The ligaments and muscles around the joint weaken and stiffen too.

Much of the risk of osteoarthritis comes from certain joints, particularly those in your knees, wrists, or fingers, being overworked from certain jobs or sports activities. If your job requires you to work in a kneeling or squatting position, for example, you might be at risk for OA in your knee. The same goes for repetitive motions like typing; this might lead to OA in your hands. To prevent this, consider creating an ergonomic work environment, using dictation programs or devices to do the typing for you, and for a positive change, instead of writing an email to a colleague, get up and walk down to his or her office (and the bonus is a little bit of exercise).

Other risk factors for OA include heredity and being overweight (which puts damaging pressure on your joints).

LIGHTEN YOUR LOAD!

The American Chiropractic Association takes issue with your oversized totes, weighted-down briefcases, and massive handbags. They may be in fashion, but if they're tipping the scales at more than 10 percent of your body weight, they should be out of the question. The long-term effects on your skeleton aren't so hip. I'm talking loss of balance, decrease in spinal health, curvature of the spine, chronic headaches, backaches, and increased risk of injury.

Remember: If you're a 150-pound woman, that purse you're slinging over your shoulder needs to weigh less than 15 pounds. After all, do you *really* need the makeup bags, bottles of water, reading material, and all the other junk you stuff in there every day? If your answer is yes, then consider a rolling bag!

The Anti-Aging Essentials and Your Musculoskeletal System

#1: Movement. When it comes to preventing injury and preserving the health and vitality of your bones, muscles, and ligaments, this should be your number-one priority. It's a recurring theme in this chapter, and you'll learn about specific moves and exercises that maximize your exercise time and have positive effects on your whole musculoskeletal system.

#2: Maintain a healthy weight. With all the movin' and groovin' you'll be doing, you're sure to lose weight and maintain that lower weight. You'll enjoy so many great benefits of weight loss, including putting less stress on your joints (like your knees) and lower levels of inflammation (which can lead to arthritis). Who wants to be stiff, achy, and cracking with every step when they're pushing 100 years old? Not you!

#3: Stay hydrated. Proper hydration helps lubricate the joints. When it comes to the knee joint, friction is the enemy, because that can cause cartilage to break down. Water helps the joints glide smoothly. But bones aren't the only benefactors: Muscles crave water too. In fact, they're mostly made of H_2O! So, drink up for strong bones and healthy muscles.

#4: Avoid smoking. Smoking can lead to bone breaks later in life because the toxins in the smoke weaken the overall bone structure by limiting the blood supply to the bones, which they desperately need in order to continue their process of building and strengthening over time. Plus, smoking keeps your body from being able to absorb calcium properly from your food. If you're a nonsmoker or have recently decided to quit, kudos! Your bones are thanking you.

#5: Supplements. Refer to my list for the specific supplements that support your musculoskeletal system . . . especially calcium!

The Number-One Strategy:
Get Movin'

You work out to stay trim, lose weight, or keep your heart up to snuff, but have you considered exercising for the sake of your musculoskeletal system? Well, you should, because exercise has near-miraculous effects on this system. It builds muscle, strengthens bones, and protects your joints.

Exercise develops muscle tissue by tearing it down and rebuilding it—in essence, stressing it. During the tear-down part of this process, "satellite" cells outside muscle tissue divide and replicate themselves. Then they fuse together and bond with the damaged muscle fibers to repair them, just as you'd repair something with Superglue. After the repair is completed, the muscle tissue is bigger and stronger than before.

With exercise—particularly strength training—your bones respond in a similar way. They get bigger and stronger because you're placing stress on them. Like muscle, bones adapt to that stress by becoming stronger. At the cellular level, bone cells multiply and manufacture new bone. That's why exercise is one of the best ways to prevent osteoporosis.

Exercise can also protect your joints, which means protection against osteoarthritis. Exercise keeps your joints flexible so you can move them through a fuller range of motion. It's like WD40 for your joints!

Exercise ultimately relieves joint pain, too. The more muscle you can build around a joint, the more support you give it, so there's less work for the joint to do. More muscle helps build balance and stability and prevent falls.

Basically, exercise fixes nearly everything that goes wrong with this system. Being active is the way we were meant to live. Not only will exercise help you move better, but you'll sleep better, eat better, and get sick less often once you take an exercise regimen seriously.

So, please: Exercise most days of the week, and exercise vigorously. It will help you live 100 happy, healthy years.

SUPPLEMENTS THAT SUPPORT YOUR MUSCULOSKELETAL SYSTEM

- **Calcium:** 1,000 mg daily
- **Vitamin D:** 800–1,000 IU daily

Why: If you aim to have enough pep in your step to play ball with your grandkids someday, you need to feed your body the nutrients it needs for muscle and bone health. Calcium supports your bones. Think of it as cement—it actually hardens your bones and keeps them strong. If you don't get enough calcium over time, you could put yourself at a higher risk of your bones breaking down and becoming brittle, and you may even develop osteoporosis. Vitamin D helps your body absorb the calcium you take in, so together, they're the perfect team.

Supportive Strategies for Bone Health

Get a bone test. I recommend that you think seriously about getting a bone density test, specifically a densitometry or DEXA scan, especially if you have any risk factors for osteoporosis. This test measures how much bone mass you have. Your doctor uses this test to predict your risk for bone fractures in the future. I'd like to assure you, however, that being at risk does not mean you have osteoporosis or will develop it. It simply means that you may want to take better care of your bone health.

Load up on calcium from nature. As I mentioned in the supplement section in this chapter, calcium is key to bone health, specifically to preventing bone deterioration when you're older. You want to keep your bones strong so they'll always support your movement and keep you out of a wheelchair later in life. But remember, I want you to get your vitamins first from food and use supplements as backup. Here are some of the winners in the calcium category.

High-calcium foods include

> Low-fat yogurt (8 ounces = approx. 345 mg calcium)
> Low-fat or 2% milk (1 cup = approx. 297 mg calcium)
> Low-fat cheese (particularly Swiss and mozzarella)
>   (1 ounce = approx. 200–270 mg calcium)

Sardines, with bones (3 ounces = approx. 324 mg calcium)
Soybeans (edamame) (1 cup = approx. 180 mg calcium)
Low-fat cottage cheese (1 cup = approx. 160 mg calcium)
Leafy green vegetables:
    Spinach (½ cup = approx. 130 mg calcium)
    Kale (½ cup = approx. 90 mg calcium)
    Collard greens (½ cup = approx. 74 mg calcium)
    Tofu (½ cup = approx. 253 mg calcium)
Okra (½ cup = approx. 88 mg calcium)

Remember, you're aiming for 1,000 milligrams daily, so if you eat a cup of low-fat yogurt, two servings of spinach, a cup of edamame, and a glass of low-fat milk, then you've met your goal.

Prevent falls. This is critical, especially as you get older! Avoid medications that cause drowsiness and remove household hazards (including throw rugs) to reduce the risk of fractures. Wear glasses or contacts if your vision isn't great. Other ways to prevent falling include the following:

Don't walk alone on icy or rainy days.
Use bars in your bathtub, when needed.
Hold onto railings when going up and down stairs.
Wear well-fitting shoes.
Make sure your home is well lit.

Medical treatments. Your doctor may put you on bisphosphonates to prevent and treat osteoporosis. Oral bisphosphonates include alendronate (Fosamax), ibandronate (Boniva), and risedronate (Actonel). Another option is calcitonin; it slows the rate of bone loss and relieves bone pain. It comes as a nasal spray or injection. The main side effects are nasal irritation from the spray form and nausea from the injectable form. Raloxifene (Evista) is also used for the prevention and treatment of osteoporosis. It can reduce the risk of spinal fractures by almost 40 percent. But it doesn't appear to prevent other fractures, including those in the hip.

Exercise. These specific types of exercises are important for strengthening bones but also establishing muscle tone and creating a synergy between all the elements of the musculoskeletal system: ligaments, bones, muscles, etc.

- *Weight-bearing exercises*—strength training, Pilates, walking, jogging, playing tennis, and dancing. These exercises help increase healthy stress on bone, thus stimulating the production of new bone cells.

- *Balance exercises*—tai chi, yoga. Both yoga and tai chi move your limbs through a wide range of motion, and this increases flexibility. Balancing moves and postures are also incorporated; some require balancing on one leg, for example. Thus, the slow, fluid movements of these exercises work muscles and improve balance and agility.

- *Cardio*—Cardio exercise, such as walking fast, jogging, biking, or rowing, has been shown to shore up bone mass in the lower spine and hip region. It enhances your heart and lung health, too, plus helps burn fat and control weight.

LADIES: HOLD THE HEELS!

It all comes down to a good pair of shoes when creating a stable foundation for your musculoskeletal system. How many times have you complained that high heels just kill your feet? You're not alone. According to the American Academy of Orthopaedic Surgeons, eight out of 10 women surveyed said their shoes cause pain. Well, that pain is your feet telling you to give them a break! Shoes that don't fit correctly or cause undue pain are major reasons for the nearly $2 billion spent by patients every year to have corrective foot surgery. Do you want to land in the category of seven out of 10 women who suffer with some kind of foot deformity, such as hammertoe or bunions? I know sometimes you think beauty requires pain, but is it really worth women being nine times more prone to foot troubles than men?

Wearing a pair of comfy kicks is a big step toward preventing injury and chronic pain to your musculoskeletal system. So, for this 17 Day Plan, hold the heels and slip into sneakers, boots, slippers, or sandals. Pick something that fits, feels comfortable, and offers support. I'm sure you don't mind having another excuse to go shoe shopping, right?

Supportive Strategies for Osteoarthritis

If I x-rayed everyone's joints after they reach age 65 or older, most patients would have some osteoarthritis. If the condition strikes you, you'll usually notice pain in your knee, hip, hand, or spine after you hit middle age. Your joints may feel stiff, too, and hard to move through a full range of motion. If you've got OA in your hip, it may be difficult to move around. If it's in your knee, your knee may give out or buckle when you walk. Back pain may be a sign of OA in your spine. Fortunately, there's a lot you can do to prevent it or keep it from worsening. Here are some important strategies.

Watch your weight. Achieve and stay at a healthy weight. This is the number-one preventive strategy for avoiding OA in your knees, hips, and spine. Use exercise to help you maintain a healthy weight. Exercise can also minimize pain, increase muscle strength, and improve flexibility.

Control pain. Apply heat or cold compresses if you have joint pain. Cold numbs the affected area, giving pain relief. Heat relaxes the muscles and relieves achy joints. Try anti-inflammatory medications. I recommend acetaminophen (Tylenol) first, because it has fewer side effects than other drugs. If your pain continues, your doctor may recommend other non-steroidal anti-inflammatory drugs (NSAIDs). Common NSAIDs include aspirin, ibuprofen, and naproxen.

But beware: Some of these medications can have some nasty side effects, such as intestinal bleeding or kidney damage. Should a joint be severely damaged, your doctor might want to inject steroids into the joint to give you relief. A more natural treatment is supplementation with glucosamine sulfate (a dietary supplement). It is both safe and effective for OA symptoms. Another is to apply a cream like Zostrix, which contains capsaicin, a natural painkiller. Capsaicin blocks the ability to feel pain, without causing numbness. It works in two ways: first, by depleting nerve cells of "substance P," a chemical messenger that relays pain sensations to the central nervous system; and second, by increasing blood flow to the area stricken with pain (increased blood flow is one of the chief ways the body heals itself).

Supportive Strategies for Muscle Health

Strength training. Strong, defined muscles not only help you chisel a nice physique, they also protect your bones and help prevent them from breaking. So if you do resistance training, you're in luck. Resistance training stimulates the formation of bone. It also improves strength and balance, which means you're less likely to risk falls and fractures.

I often emphasize to patients that the all-time best "therapy" for muscle health and fitness is resistance training—exercise that increases muscle strength and endurance with weights or resistance bands. If you're new to strength training, your best bet is to work your body three days a week, on nonconsecutive days. This schedule gives your body time to rest so that it can respond by increasing bone and muscle strength. If you've never done strength training a day in your life, let me encourage you to work with a qualified personal trainer who can show you the ropes. You need to master the basics before moving on to more intense weight-lifting.

I recommend focusing on four exercise patterns:

- **Push against resistance.** Do exercises that involve pushing, such as push-ups, to challenge your triceps, chest, and shoulders.
- **Pull.** Pulling exercises, such as chin-ups, biceps curls, and rowing, target the upper back, the back of the shoulders, and the biceps.
- **Work your legs.** A bunch of exercises, including leg extensions, squats, lunges, climbing stairs, and jumping up and down, can improve strength in your upper and lower legs.
- **Build your core.** Exercises such as sit-ups, crunches, and twisting motions focus on the core muscles of the abdomen and back. Core strength preserves mobility and protects your back muscles.

Protein. There's a lot of hype about high-protein diets out there, so I'm going to make this very simple. Women, on average, require about 46 grams of protein daily, and men require about 56 grams. That means 10 to 35 percent of your daily calories should come from protein.

High-protein foods include

- Tuna (3 oz.)—about 22 grams protein
- Lean beef steak (4 oz.)—about 23 grams protein
- Chicken breast (3 oz.)—about 21 grams protein
- Shrimp (3 oz.)—about 18 grams protein
- One cup of beans (dry beans)—about 16 grams protein
- One 8-ounce cup of nonfat Greek yogurt—about 11 grams protein
- One glass of 2% milk—about 8 grams protein
- One whole egg—about 7 grams protein
- One egg white—about 4 grams protein

So, does your daily diet provide you with enough protein without packing in extra fat grams? If not, consider a whey protein shake after your workouts or first thing in the morning. Experts believe whey protein is the most "bioavailable" of all the protein supplements; it is fast absorbing and highly digestible in your body. But don't overdo it, because there's no benefit to exceeding the recommended daily dose of protein unless you are an athlete, or in training.

Before you begin the Cycle 2: 17 Day Plan, I want you to take this quiz and score yourself. Then, take the quiz again after you've completed the 17 days for proof of your improvement.

Is Your Musculoskeletal System on Its Way to 100 Happy, Healthy Years?

Read each question carefully and select your answer. Add up your points and see how you scored.

---

1. **How many push-ups can you complete in 60 seconds? Do them on your knees, if you need to.**

     A. 10 or fewer ☐ 0 points
     B. 11 to 15 ☐ 1 point
     C. 16 to 20 ☐ 2 points
     D. 21 to 30 ☐ 3 points
     E. More than 30 ☐ 4 points

2. **Can you raise your arms fully above your head, using resistance (such as a set of 5- to 10-pound dumbbells)?**

   A. No ☐ 0 points
   B. Only partway ☐ 2 points
   C. Yes ☐ 4 points

3. **How far forward can you bend at your waist?**

   A. I can barely bend. ☐ 0 points
   B. I can bend about halfway. ☐ 2 points
   C. I can bend as far as to touch my knees. ☐ 3 points
   D. I can bend forward and touch my fingers or hands to the floor.
      ☐ 4 points

4. **Has anyone in your family ever been diagnosed with osteoporosis?**

   A. Yes ☐ immediate family, including grandparents ☐ 0 points
   B. Yes ☐ more distant relatives, such as cousins or aunts
      ☐ 2 points
   C. No, or not to my knowledge ☐ 4 points

5. **Are you a smoker?**

   A. Yes, I smoke regularly. ☐ 0 points
   B. Sometimes, at social events or on the weekend. ☐ 1 point
   C. I'm in the process of quitting. ☐ 2 points
   D. No ☐ 4 points

6. **What is the total number of alcoholic beverages you consume, on average, per day?**

   A. Three or more drinks ☐ 0 points
   B. Two drinks ☐ 2 points
   C. None to one drink ☐ 4 points

7. **How many total cups of caffeinated beverages (coffee, soda, or tea) do you consume in a week?**

   A. More than 14 ☐ 0 points
   B. Seven to 14 ☐ 2 points
   C. None to six ☐ 4 points

8. **How much (and what type of) exercise do you get on average?**

   A. None ☐ 0 points
   B. Gentle exercises like yoga, tai chi, or swimming, two or three days a week ☐ 2 points
   C. Activities like walking, running, ball sports, or weight training, at least three days a week ☐ 4 points

9. **Do you eat dairy products or take calcium supplements?**

   A. No ☐ 0 points
   B. Yes, every now and again ☐ 1 point
   C. Yes, at least once a day ☐ 4 points

10. **Are you spending, on average, 10 or more minutes outdoors every day?**

    A. No, I avoid the sun whenever I can. ☐ 0 points
    B. Only in the summer, when the weather is warm ☐ 2 points
    C. Yes, at least 10 minutes on most days ☐ 4 points

11. **Are you currently overweight?**

    A. Yes, and I'm not actively trying to lose weight. ☐ 0 points
    B. Yes, but I'm on a program to lose the weight. ☐ 2 points
    C. No, I'm not overweight. ☐ 4 points

12. **Do you consume, on average, 46 grams of protein daily if you're a woman, or 56 grams of protein daily if you're a man?**

    A. No ☐ 0 points   B. Yes ☐ 4 points

13. **Do you currently have arthritis, or a family history of arthritis?**

    A. Yes, and I'm not taking anything for it. ☐ 0 points
    B. Yes, but I'm on supplements or medication to help.
       ☐ 2 points
    C. No ☐ 4 points

14. **How often do you wear high heels?**

    A. Very often ☐ 0 points
    B. Sometimes ☐ 2 points
    C. Rarely ☐ 3 points
    D. Never ☐ 4 points

How you move, groove, run, jump, and walk all depend on the biggest system in your body—the musculoskeletal system. I want you to glide right into your latter years, head held high, back straight, and even with a confident swagger. Put a little effort into protecting your precious bones, muscles, ligaments, tendons, and joints now and reap the wheelchair-free benefits later.

CHAPTER 11

Cycle 2: 17 Day Plan

In Cycle 1: Restore, we focused on getting your primary systems up to snuff and at a baseline level of health. Isn't it remarkable how simple changes in your daily life can make such big differences?

If you feel you have more work to do on the Cycle 1 systems, don't worry, because we're not abandoning them in Cycle 2: Rebuild. Since all of your body's systems are interrelated, what benefits one system simultaneously boosts another. Plus, you will alternate your Restore days with Rebuild days. In other words, you'll continue restoring the health of your heart, lungs, and brain while you're rebuilding and strengthening your supportive systems.

Cycle 2: Rebuild targets the immune, digestive, endocrine, and musculoskeletal systems. You are working toward bolstering their health so you can function at your highest level—now and down the road. Here's what I mean:

Goals of Cycle 2: Rebuild

Increase your resistance against illness
Improve how you feel overall
Sleep better
Reduce any digestive symptoms (constipation, acid reflux, etc.)
Enhance nutrient absorption
Boost your metabolism
Maintain and/or boost thyroid function
Reduce stress
Prevent osteoporosis or slow it down
Build muscle to augment calorie burn
Alleviate and prevent joint pain

These may seem like lofty goals, but again, you'll be surprised by how small adjustments in your day-to-day activities will do big favors for these systems, and ultimately, for your overall health and well-being. There are a few things to keep in mind on a daily basis throughout Cycle 2: Rebuild.

Before Beginning Cycle 2

1. Conduct a thorough kitchen clean-out. Remove all packaged, processed, and sugary junk foods. No excuses about your cousin coming to visit from out of town in a few weeks or whatever nonsense you're telling yourself for why you simply can't get rid of this stuff. Get it all out!

2. Your next stop is the grocery store. Stock up on colorful fruits and vegetables in their natural form, as well as other healthy, unprocessed foods.

3. Make sure you're taking 1,200 milligrams of calcium and 800 to 1,000 IU (international units) of vitamin D. You'll probably have to take these as two separate supplements.

4. Purchase a probiotic and a zinc supplement. Take them every morning with your multivitamin. Instead of a probiotic in pill or powder form, you can eat one serving of low-fat yogurt with live active cultures each day on the plan.

5. **Arthritis sufferers:** If your doctor has recommended or approved of you taking glucosamine and chondroitin supplements, be sure to take the recommended dosage on the bottle every day.

General Guidelines for Cycle 2: Rebuild

1. Try going to bed and getting up at the same time every day on this plan. This reinforces your body's circadian rhythms, or natural sleep cycles, and promotes deeper sleep. Regular sleep like this will allow your immune system to reset each night so it can do its hardest work for you.

2. Thoroughly wash your hands with soap and water frequently throughout each day on this plan, especially after you shake

hands with someone, touch something in public, or use the rest-room and before you prepare food or eat. Preventing the spread of germs before they can enter your body is a key to not getting sick. You should also consider carrying hand sanitizer with you at all times.

3. Call your doctor(s) and make appointments if any of these apply to you:

    • You aren't up to date on any of your adult booster vaccines.

    • You are due for a mammogram.

    • You are due for a bone scan.

    • You are experiencing any new symptoms (including lethargy).

    • If you're not sure when you're due for any of these items, it's as simple as making a phone call to find out. Poor record-keeping doesn't get you off the hook!

4. Spend at least 10 minutes outside each day. Soak up some sunshine so your body can naturally produce vitamin D. (I admit, I live in California where the sun shines quite often. I get that this isn't feasible for everyone on a daily basis during winter, but there are three other seasons in which this certainly holds true.)

5. Find ways to increase your NEAT (nonexercise activity thermogenesis) each day on this cycle. Here are some examples:

    • Stand up and pace while you're on the phone.

    • Walk to destinations.

    • Park farther away from stores.

    • Climb the stairs instead of taking the elevator.

    • Clean your house vigorously.

    • Stand while you fold the laundry.

    • Rake the lawn.

    • Do a walk-and-talk meeting.

6. In addition to your NEAT, work in 30 minutes of continuous cardio-vascular exercise each day. Work to get in your *cardio zone* but not above it. You can find out how to calculate your cardio zone in the Appendix.

- You will also find many exercises designed to boost the health of your musculoskeletal system in this plan. The options and descriptions of these exercises can also be found in the Appendix.

7. **Overall food choices:** Commit to yourself that for the next 17 days (it's not that long!) you will do the following:

   - **No white:** Remove from your diet all "white" foods such as refined sugar (including soda and sweets), white bread, pasta made with white flour (whole wheat is okay), and other foods made with white flour.

   - **Whole foods:** Eat all of your foods as close to their whole, natural state as possible.

   - **Balanced plate:** Make sure approximately one-third of your calories come from lean protein, which is the healthiest balance for your endocrine system.

   - **Fiber:** Eat your recommended amount of fiber each day (try some of my FFFs!):

     - Women under 50: 25 grams of fiber daily
     - Women over 50: 21 grams of fiber daily
     - Men under 50: 38 grams of fiber daily
     - Men over 50: 30 grams of fiber daily

8. Take the following supplements, which are also mentioned in the previous chapters. But check your multivitamin to make sure you aren't doubling up on anything:

   - Zinc: 11 mg daily for men, 8 mg daily for women
   - Vitamin C: 1,000 mg daily
   - Folic acid: .4 mg daily
   - Ginseng: as directed
   - Probiotics: One to 10 billion CFU (colony-forming units) or living organisms. Take dosage recommended on the bottle, since they differ. Alternatively, eat one serving of low-fat yogurt with live active cultures daily.
   - Vitamin D: 800 to 1,000 IU daily

- Vitamin E: 15 mg daily
- Selenium: 55 mcg daily
- Calcium: 1,000 mg daily
- Green tea: One cup daily

9. Become mindful of your eating habits. Don't eat with the TV on. Chew slowly, put the fork down between bites, and avoid drinking liquid during each meal so you don't wash away precious nutrients you're consuming in the foods.

10. Purchase or make seaweed snacks to enjoy periodically during this cycle, not only for the iodine they provide for your thyroid, but also because they are a low-cal, nutrient-dense snack. If you don't like them (though I find them delicious), consume several servings of other iodine-rich foods like shellfish, radishes, or parsley instead.

11. A few hours before bed each night on this plan, I encourage you to rate your stress level on a scale of 1 to 10 and write it down. Are you at a 5 or above? If so, record what's stressing you out on a stress chart. Begin thinking of solutions for dealing with these details. Take two minutes to breathe deeply, letting the stress out with each exhale. Commit to relaxing the rest of each evening before going to bed. This procedure will go a long way toward helping you learn to manage the manageable stress in your life.

12. Limit, or better yet, eliminate alcohol from your diet during this cycle. It's only 17 days; you can do it! This will ease your digestion and reduce your overall sugar intake, which improves immunity and allows your body to better absorb calcium for strong bones.

Day 1

Upon rising: Perform 10 minutes of *pull exercises* of your choice.

Breakfast: Include one food high in calcium and one fruit high in antioxidants.

- *Idea:* Eat eight ounces of low-fat yogurt sprinkled with cinnamon for extra flavor, and one handful of any berries.

All day: Don't blast the air conditioner or heater in your car, home, or office. Let your body do the work to keep you cool or warm. This kicks your endocrine system and metabolism into a higher gear.

Lunch: Include at least one food high in selenium.

- *Examples:* Cod, turkey, tuna, halibut, mushrooms, sunflower seeds, Brazil nuts, barley.
- *Idea:* Sprinkle sunflower seeds and chopped mushrooms in a spinach salad.

Midday: Perform *stork stance* for two minutes to challenge your balance, strengthen bones, and prevent falls later in life.

Dinner: Prepare your lean protein in two teaspoons of coconut oil instead of your regular cooking oil.

- Remember, switching up the types of fats in cooking oils can help prevent type 2 diabetes down the line.

Evening: Laugh out loud for 10 minutes to increase circulation and thus immunity.

- *Idea:* Watch funny YouTube videos or do *Laughter Yoga*.

Day 2

Follow **Restore Cycle** Day 2.

Day 3

Upon rising: Perform *push exercises* of your choice for 10 minutes.

Breakfast: Include one food high in calcium and one fruit high in antioxidants.

- *Idea:* Eat one slice of low-fat cheese with two egg whites and a handful of any berries.

Lunch: Include at least one food high in antioxidants.

Midday: Take a spirulina supplement (or one serving of spirulina powder in a smoothie) and have one high-calcium food as a snack.

Evening: Prepare a double batch of *Dr. Mike's Mashed Un-Potatoes*, and portion them out into containers. Snack on them through the rest of the week!

Dinner: Include at least one food high in beta-carotene or other antioxidants, but keep it as close to its natural form as possible.

- *Idea:* Chop up asparagus and bell peppers and quickly sauté them so they maintain a nice crunch.

Day 4

Follow **Restore Cycle** Day 4.

Day 5

Upon rising: Perform *pull exercises* of your choice for 10 minutes.

All day: Don't blast your air conditioner or heater in your car, home, or office. Let your body do the work to keep you cool or warm.

Breakfast: Include one food high in calcium and one fruit high in antioxidants.

- *Idea:* Eat eight ounces of low-fat cottage cheese and one apricot.

Anytime: During your cardiovascular workout, perform 10 *butt kickers* on each side.

Lunch: Include at least one food high in antioxidants.

- *Idea:* Enjoy some of the *Dr. Mike's Mashed Un-Potatoes* with your lean protein.

Midday: Take a spirulina supplement, or put a scoop of spirulina powder in a protein shake.

Dinner: Work in at least one food high in selenium.

- *Idea:* Make homemade fish tacos with cod or halibut, and sprinkle a few sunflower seeds on top!

Evening: Laugh out loud for 10 minutes.

Day 6

Follow **Restore Cycle** Day 6.

Day 7

Upon rising: Perform 10 minutes of *leg exercises* of your choice.

- Building strong quadriceps and other leg muscles helps prevent knee and hip pain later in life.

Breakfast: Include one food high in calcium and one fruit high in anti-oxidants.

All day: Don't blast your air conditioner or heater in your car, home, or office. Let your body do the work to keep you cool or warm.

Midday: Take a spirulina supplement, or put a scoop of spirulina powder in a protein shake.

Lunch: Include at least one food high in antioxidants, specifically beta-carotene.

After lunch: Drink a glass of ice-cold water for a midday metabolism boost.

Dinner: Work in at least one food high in selenium and prepare your lean protein using coconut oil.

Before bed: When you're washing your face, give yourself a one-minute facial and neck massage. Target your lymph nodes, and move your fingers down, encouraging the lymph to drain.

Day 8

Follow **Restore Cycle** Day 8.

Day 9

Breakfast: Include one food high in calcium and one fruit high in antioxidants.

- *Idea:* Eat a bowl of low-sugar, high-fiber cereal with ½ cup of low-fat milk, plus a generous handful of blackberries on top.

Mid-morning: Do four sets of *core exercises* of your choice.

Lunch: Include at least one food high in antioxidants.

Midday: Exercise your ankles by performing two minutes of *ankle circles*. These will help prevent ankle injuries during workouts and everyday life.

Dinner: Work in at least one food high in selenium.

- Remember, there's enough selenium in one Brazil nut to get your entire day's dose.

Day 10

Follow **Restore Cycle** Day 10.

Day 11

Anytime: During your cardiovascular workout, perform 10 *butt kickers* on each side.

Breakfast: Include one food high in calcium and one fruit high in antioxidants.

Lunch: Include at least one food high in antioxidants.

Midday: Take a spirulina supplement, or put a scoop of spirulina powder in a protein shake.

Late afternoon: Drink a glass of ice water for a boost to your metabolism.

Evening: Prepare another double batch of *Dr. Mike's Mashed Un-Potatoes* and portion it out into containers. Snack on them through the rest of the week!

Dinner: Include at least one food high in selenium.

Day 12

Follow **Restore Cycle** Day 12.

Day 13

Upon rising: Perform 10 minutes of *leg exercises* of your choice and 10 minutes of *push exercises*.

Breakfast: Include one food high in calcium and one fruit high in antioxidants.

All day: Don't blast your air conditioner or heater in your car, home, or office. Let your body do the work to keep you cool or warm.

Midday: Take a spirulina supplement, or put a scoop of spirulina powder in a protein shake.

Dinner: Work in at least one food high in selenium.

Evening: Perform one *balance exercise* of your choice for five minutes.

Day 14

Follow **Restore Cycle** Day 14.

Day 15

All day: Don't blast your air conditioner or heater in your car, home, or office. Let your body do the work to keep you cool or warm.

Breakfast: Include one food high in calcium and one fruit high in antioxidants.

Midday: Take a spirulina supplement, or put a scoop of spirulina powder in a protein shake.

Afternoon snack: Have a selenium snack such as a tablespoon of sunflower seeds.

Dinner: Work in at least one food high in beta-carotene.

Evening: Just before your cardiovascular workout tonight, do two minutes of *arm circles*, changing direction every 20 seconds.

Before bed: When you're washing your face, give yourself a one-minute facial and neck massage. Target your lymph nodes, and move your fingers down, encouraging the lymph to drain.

Day 16

Follow **Restore Cycle** Day 16.

Day 17

Upon rising: Perform 10 minutes of *pull exercises* of your choice.

Breakfast: Include a handful of berries (strawberries, blueberries, blackberries) in your oatmeal or protein shake.

Mid-morning: Do two sets of the *executive stretches* and four sets of *core exercises*.

Lunch: Include at least one food high in selenium. *Examples:* cod, turkey, tuna, halibut, mushrooms, sunflower seeds, Brazil nuts, barley.

Midday: Take a spirulina supplement, or put a scoop of spirulina powder in a protein shake.

Dinner: Work in at least one food high in selenium.

Evening: Laugh out loud for at least 10 minutes. Do whatever it takes to get a good, long giggling session going!

Before bed: When you're washing your face, give yourself a one-minute facial and neck massage. Target your lymph nodes, and move your fingers down, encouraging the lymph to drain.

You've completed the Cycle 2: Rebuild—how do you feel? My guess is that you're ready to race the Energizer bunny and leap over tall buildings. You've just taken yourself into a whole new fat-burning zone by boosting your metabolism, quickened your overall immune response to invaders, toned and shaped your supportive muscles, and built stronger bones—all in just 17 days. Not to mention that I bet you're more rested than you've been in quite some time! The habits are such simple ones to adopt, and I encourage you to continue them going forward.

It's time to continue our journey toward a lifetime of good health and happiness with Cycle 3: Refine. Let's carry on!

PART FOUR

●●●●●●●●●●●●●●●●●●●●●●●●●●●●

Cycle 3: Refine

In Cycle 3: Refine, we'll turn our focus toward the delicate reproductive and urinary systems. Just like the systems we've explored so far, these three are highly susceptible to the five factors of aging. In order to stop or reverse their decline and to protect your overall health as you march toward your future, it's important that you understand their roles and how to strengthen them.

After all, don't you want to do everything you can to prevent incontinence in your old age? How about helping your body burn calories and fat so you can avoid that midlife spare-tire effect?

I'll also give you the tools you need to reduce the risk of illnesses associated with the reproductive system as you get older. Ladies, did you ever think menopause could be cause for celebration? I'll tell you why, and I'll help you understand your options better than ever before. Men: You will also find a chapter specifically targeted at enhancing the function of the male reproductive system as you get older. This includes all the insider secrets to postponing or reversing the effects of andropause, or what some people begrudgingly refer to as "man-o-pause."

Listen, I want you to love and enjoy life more and

more as you turn the pages of your calendar. I have a passion for helping people become and remain healthy enough to live out their dreams. You may have to make some changes, but they'll be worth it. I can hardly wait for you to get started!

CHAPTER 12

Still Sexy After All Those Years

Yes, ladies, the verdict is in: Older women are officially declared sexy. Look around you . . . the role models of fabulous women over the age of 50 abound, particularly in the media: Diane Keaton, Michelle Pfeiffer, and Angela Bassett, to name just a few. And the "cougars" are getting a lot of attention these days as younger men vie for their attention. Will you age like these beauties, or will you spend your golden years reminiscing about how once upon a time you were young and vibrant? I'm sure you'll opt for the former, so I'll help you get there. Getting older can definitely be sexy if you follow my advice. Here we go, starting with a little anatomy lesson about your reproductive system, one of the sources of your sexiness and femininity.

The Female Reproductive System 101

The organs that make up your reproductive system include the ovaries, uterus, and vagina, and they all take on roles that go beyond their basic functions. Take the ovaries, for example. While the ovaries are responsible for producing eggs and keeping your menstrual cycle in good working order, they are also responsible for secreting hormones that help you feel and look good during your childbearing years. The uterus carries and nurtures your developing baby, and if it is your desire, fulfills your need for becoming a mom. The vagina accepts sperm, and is the pathway for the baby's entry into the world. Of course it is a sexual organ, too, with its many nerve endings to bring you pleasure during intimacy.

All of these organs change with age, and, understandably, these changes can affect your sense of self. Your ovaries and vagina shrink at menopause. Your vagina may quit lubricating, and your sexual desire might wane as a result. You might need to have your uterus or organs removed for medical and health reasons. But it's not all bad news—far from it. In my practice, I've seen women who keep themselves in good health, their bodies in great shape, and have a realistic, positive attitude toward these changes. The result is a satisfying sex life, a vibrant, healthy life, and a joie de vivre well into their golden years. In this chapter, I'm going to help you join that still-sexy sorority.

So let's start in the middle of your life—with menopause. Even if you're aware of wrinkles popping up or gray hair taking over long before you hit middle age, this is the time when you might realize more profoundly that getting older is unavoidable.

How Your Reproductive System Ages

Women, your reproductive system will gradually age and it may do so in many different ways, from the natural (like menopause) to the unnatural (like cancer). Before I get into specific strategies for postponing or improving your experience with these, let me talk to you about the single most important factor of aging over which you have control, and that is halting oxidative stress. If you remember, oxidative stress occurs when cell-damaging free radicals outnumber protective antioxidants. So you want to be doing everything I've noted to prevent oxidative stress: Take supplemental antioxidants, eat colorful, antioxidant-rich foods, exercise, and keep your weight under control because obesity increases oxidative stress and heightens the risk of female cancer. Another strategy for combating oxidative stress is to consider hormone replacement therapy (HRT) after you hit menopause. That's because oxidative stress in a woman's body increases after menopause, and estrogen-only replacement therapy can help prevent it. Speaking of menopause, let's talk about how to handle this inevitable stage of life in a way that will help you stay young and vibrant on your way to 100 happy, healthy years.

SUPPLEMENTS THAT SUPPORT YOUR FEMALE REPRODUCTIVE SYSTEM

- **Vitamin E—400 IU daily (do not exceed)**

  Why: Vitamin E has been found to reduce symptoms of both PMS and menopause because it can reduce your body's production of prostaglandins, which are substances similar to hormones known to cause cramps and breast tenderness.

However, do not exceed the recommended daily dose of vitamin E, because too much of it can lead to blood-clotting problems and increase the risk of stroke.

SEVEN REASONS TO TALK TO YOUR DOC ABOUT HORMONE REPLACEMENT THERAPY (HRT)

1. You're suffering really miserable menopause symptoms such as hot flashes or insomnia.
2. You want to juice up your libido. (HRT increases sex drive and lubricates your nether regions for more satisfying sex.)
3. You're at risk of osteoporosis. (HRT lowers that risk.)
4. You're concerned about heart disease. Harvard research tells us that women who go on HRT soon after starting menopause have a 30 percent lower risk of heart disease than those who never went on hormones.
5. You're at risk of colon cancer (it runs in your family, or you've had polyps in your colon in the past).
6. You're having problems with incontinence. (Estrogen helps prevent it.)
7. You wouldn't mind having younger-looking skin. (Experts believe estrogen helps prevent your skin from aging.)

HRT involves taking estrogen, sometimes in combination with progesterone. It can treat most symptoms of menopause: severe hot flashes, night sweats, mood issues, and vaginal dryness. It is a great option for many women, but if you go this route, your physician should monitor you regularly. First, you should have a hormone panel (a type of blood test) done so you know exactly which hormones you're deficient in. There are various types and methods of HRT (including pills, patches, creams, vaginal rings, tablets, etc.), so make the decision with your doctor about which form is right for you.

Some experts believe HRT could increase women's breast cancer risks, so especially if you have a family history of breast or ovarian cancer, discuss those factors with your gynecologist.

As you plan for menopause and make decisions with your gynecologist about hormone replacement therapy, bring up any concerns you have about your risk for breast cancer. Be sure to share information about family history and go over all the potential factors at play before you start your HRT. If you're already on any type of estrogen or progesterone treatments, talk to your doctor about whether you should make any changes to your current plan to avoid increasing your odds of a breast cancer diagnosis later on.

The Anti-Aging Essentials and Your Reproductive System

#1: Movement. No matter where you are in your reproductive life—from just starting menstruation to entering menopause and beyond—daily movement has a positive effect on all parts of your reproductive system. For example, women with a sedentary lifestyle are at higher risk for infertility. Studies show that menopausal women who work out regularly typically have less belly fat and naturally increased estrogen levels. Plus, hitting the gym can help cool down hot flashes. Scientists aren't exactly sure why, but they speculate that working out makes you feel so good that you can better handle troublesome menopausal symptoms.

#2: Maintain a healthy weight. As your metabolism naturally slows over time, weight gain has a way of sneaking up on you. Being overweight increases your odds of getting breast cancer, and gaining the weight later in life escalates the risk even more. Both overweight women and underweight women are more likely to experience irregular menstrual periods or cycles. Overweight women also may experience an increased risk of infertility. Furthermore, being obese or overweight puts you at risk for polycystic ovary syndrome (PCOS), which means your sex hormones are out of balance. All of this is reversible by getting into a healthy weight range. You don't need to weigh yourself every day, but pick one morning per week that you jump on the scale, completely naked, as soon as you wake up (and after you pee). Take notice of any gain, and remember that even a pound here or there can gradually add up. Adjust your diet and exercise routines accordingly to keep a consistent, healthy weight.

#3: Stay hydrated. Drinking enough water is vital to your natural vaginal lubrication. Also, it's especially important to stay hydrated when you have your period, due to the fluid you're losing.

#4: Avoid smoking. All of the responsibilities and structures of your reproductive system—from the ones involved in menstruation to ovulation to birth—are impacted negatively by tobacco use. Smoking increases your odds of infertility, preterm delivery, stillbirth, and birth defects. One study even shows that smokers may experience an earlier onset of menopause.

#5: Supplements. Keep taking that multivitamin every day and refer to my list for the specifics supplements that support your reproductive system.

Menopause

Technically, menopause marks the permanent end of menstruation and fertility, defined as occurring 12 months after your last menstrual period. It normally occurs between the ages of 45 and 55. What actually triggers menopause? It's the natural decline in your reproductive hormones, mainly estrogen. Menopause can happen naturally or in some cases surgically if you have to have your ovaries removed.

For too long in medicine, doctors and other health care practitioners have treated menopause as a disease, throwing drugs from hormones to antidepressants at women who are experiencing it. However, menopause is a natural stage of life—one that should be celebrated. At the very least you can celebrate no more cramps, no more periods, no more tampons, and even greater libido as your hormonal balance shifts to less estrogen and more testosterone (which is a natural hormonal aphrodisiac). And heck, you don't have to use contraception anymore. Menopause is a great time in your life!

However, there can be symptoms, ranging from mild to severe. This all depends on your individual makeup—and to some extent, your attitude toward menopause. A positive attitude that embraces the "Change" will help conquer the symptoms. Should you have symptoms that need easing, let me give you some strategies.

Supportive Strategies for Menopause

Consider OTC progesterone cream. If you have hot flashes or night sweats, try an over-the-counter progesterone cream. Apply it at night. These creams can work wonders and you don't even need a prescription, although I still recommend you discuss this with your gynecologist.

Have more sex. Clitoral shrinkage can occur in menopause if you're not having sex. In other words, use it or lose it! Your clitoris is filled with nerve endings and is the pivotal point in your body that stimulates you to have orgasms. Staying sexually active can also help with the vaginal dryness you may experience. Plus, more lovemaking can make you feel more sexy!

Try vaginal estrogen. For vaginal dryness, vaginal estrogen can be a great treatment. This can be administered directly to the vagina using a vaginal tablet, ring, cream, or over-the-counter lubricant. I have many patients who say they work like a charm.

Hold the heat. For some women, hot foods can set off hot flashes. I'm talking about foods and drinks that are hot temperature-wise as well as spicy ones. Alcohol can also be problematic. When you have a hot flash, think about what foods or drinks you've had recently; you'll likely start noticing a pattern that will help you figure out which foods offend you.

Unwind. Anything that calms you down can also alleviate your symptoms. So whether you enjoy meditation, massage, watching your favorite television shows, reading, or listening to music, now is the time to make relaxation a priority. Doctor's orders!

Try herbs. Consider natural herbal estrogen supplements that exist in an over-the-counter form. I have many patients who say these can really help reduce symptoms.

Consider an antidepressant. For mood swings you may experience, talk to your physician about taking an antidepressant, which boosts serotonin (a feel-good brain chemical) and can help stabilize mood.

Stay positive! Menopause doesn't mean you're old. It means you're free! It isn't just about the end of your reproductive years; it can be the beginning of a new, exciting chapter in your life. Keep a positive attitude.

Breast Cancer

While breast cancer can strike a woman—or man—of any age, advanced age is one of the risk factors for developing this disease. Women who are

55 years old or older are at a higher risk for breast cancer than younger women. In fact, two-thirds of invasive breast cancer diagnoses occur in women over 55. There's been a lot of press about certain genes called the BRCA1 or BRCA2, which have been identified as genetic mutations that put you at a greater risk of developing breast or other types of cancer. However, just having these gene mutations or a family history of breast cancer does not mean you're doomed to receive a cancer diagnosis. There are other risk factors for breast cancer, including obesity, a late-in-life pregnancy, and starting menopause at a later-than-average age. As I mentioned, some experts also believe HRT can put you at increased risk, so discuss its risks with your doctor.

Supportive Strategies for Preventing Breast Cancer

Examine your alcoholic intake. The data on this can be slightly confusing, but I'll help you sort it out. There's very strong evidence that a reasonable, modest amount of alcohol, included in an overall healthy diet and lifestyle, can help reduce the risk of stroke and heart attack. On the flip side, some convincing studies have shown that consumption of alcohol can increase your risk of breast cancer. Based on this, here is my suggestion. If you are already in a high-risk category for breast cancer due to obesity, family history, or other factors, I recommend that you truly limit your consumption of alcoholic beverages. But if you don't have several risk factors for breast cancer and you currently maintain a healthy diet and lifestyle, then it's perfectly fine to consume three to six drinks per week. Just don't drink them all at once! And don't kid yourself about your portion sizes. Just because half a bottle of wine fits in a large wineglass does not mean that's one serving. Five ounces of wine is one serving and is basically equal in alcohol content to 12 ounces of light beer or 1.5 ounces of 80-proof liquor. Sip slowly and enjoy!

PROPER SELF BREAST EXAM TECHNIQUE

I suggest you perform a self breast exam every 30 days. Here's how. Lie down on a comfortable surface. Start with your right arm extended up, behind your head. Using the index finger, middle finger, and ring finger of your left hand, inspect the right breast for lumps by pressing in small circular motions. You'll use three types of pressure for each circle: first gentle, then medium, and then firm. This way, you're able to feel for lumps at different depths within the breast tissue. You want to cover a lot of area—from your ribs (beneath your breasts) up to your clavicle—because breast tissue extends all over the chest. Experts recommend performing the exam in an up-and-down (vertical) motion, as opposed to circular, because you're more likely to cover the entire region. Repeat this process on the left breast using your right hand. Do you notice any lumps or changes that feel different from the rest of your breast, or different from what you've felt before? Do you feel something on one breast that is different from the other breast? If so, call your doctor for further examination.

The second part of the self breast exam is to stand naked in front of a mirror, place your hands on your hip bones, and visually inspect your breasts. Have they changed in any way? Any increase or decrease in overall size or volume? Has their shape changed at all? Do you notice any dimpling or changes in the skin and appearance, including the nipples?

Finally, it's imperative to inspect the area under each of your arms, but don't extend your arm straight up for this. Only bring each arm halfway up, so the skin in your armpit isn't pulled completely taut. Press with the three different pressures in the underarm area, also feeling for any new lumps or changes.

Again, if you feel or see anything abnormal, call your doctor right away to schedule an appointment for further examination. Even if you're doing self breast exams regularly, they don't replace mammograms. Talk to your doctor about when you should have a mammogram.

Atrophic Vaginitis

This is just a fancy term for extreme dryness inside the vagina. It can cause some major discomfort, especially during sex. In fact, many women experiencing atrophic vaginitis avoid intercourse altogether. The cause of this condition goes back to the decrease in estrogen caused by menopause. When estrogen decreases, tissues inside the vagina thin out, and the ability to produce lubrication naturally is hindered. Once the healthy lubrication goes away, the vagina can become irritated and inflamed, which is made worse by douching (not recommended), certain medications, soaps, and lotions. Anywhere between 10 and 40 percent of menopausal or postmenopausal women will suffer from atrophic vaginitis at some point, but many women don't think to mention it to their doctors, so the numbers may be much higher.

Supportive Strategies for Atrophic Vaginitis (Vaginal Dryness)

Don't neglect sex. Leading up to and during menopause, one of the best things you can do for your body is to have plenty of sex. Women who are more sexually active experience less vaginal dryness because they have increased blood flow to the vagina. More blood flow means the tissues stay healthier and are less likely to atrophy.

Familiarize yourself with lubricants. If you're uncomfortable shopping in "that" aisle in the grocery store, go online and order a few different types of vaginal lubricants and try them out to see which one you like the best. There are lots of options out there, and they will make a huge difference in your comfort when you're having sexual intercourse. And as I said, the more you can have sex, the healthier your vaginal tissues will remain over time.

Pelvic Organ Prolapse

As women get older, the various ligaments and muscles that hold the vagina, uterus, bladder, and lower parts of the intestines in place have a tendency to weaken and thin out. This weakening can cause those pelvic organs, especially the bladder, to drop down. It is caused by more than just gravity—childbirth can be a factor in pelvic organ prolapse, specifically vaginal childbirth. Women with multiple children tend to be at a higher risk for developing this later in life. Other causes include obesity (which adds undue pressure to this region), pelvic or back injury, chronic constipation, and other conditions that increase pressure. Too many women ignore the symptoms of pain and pressure, and let this go on far longer than they should. There are solutions! There are also ways to prevent it before it starts.

Supportive Strategies for Preventing Pelvic Organ Prolapse

Take the pressure off. Anything you can do to reduce the pressure you're putting on the pelvic region is going to help prevent the development of prolapse. This includes reaching and staying at a healthy weight, reducing any activity that leads to coughing (this includes smoking), keeping your bowels moving so you aren't constipated, and not often engaging in physical activities that strain those pelvic floor muscles too much.

Kegel exercises. You will also find this exercise in the chapter on your urinary system because it can also help prevent urinary incontinence. I encourage any woman who's had children to do these regularly because they strengthen the pelvic floor muscles. Here's how: First, to familiarize yourself with the pelvic muscles, try to stop the flow of urination halfway through. When it stops, you know you've just used the muscles we're targeting. Don't squeeze your legs, buttocks, or abdominal muscles, though. We want to isolate the pelvic floor. You'll feel a pulling sensation when you flex these muscles. Now you're ready to give them a workout! You can do this anywhere, anytime—no one will even know. Simply contract the muscles for five seconds, then release for five seconds. Repeat the process for 10 reps. You're done!

Discuss treatment with a specialist. If you're already noticing symptoms of pelvic organ prolapse, such as pressure or frequent need to urinate, you should ask your general practitioner to recommend a urogynecologist (exactly what it sounds like—a combo of a urologist and a gynecolosist) to further examine you. This specialist can offer relief, based on the type of prolapse you have. Sometimes a removable device called a pessary, which is inserted into the vagina, can stop the symptoms and keep the condition from getting any worse. In severe cases, surgery may be warranted; there have been many advances in this surgery in recent years, making it less invasive and quite successful. The bottom line is this: You don't have to live with pelvic organ prolapse, so take action and get the relief you deserve.

Endometrial Cancer

Sometimes referred to as uterine cancer, endometrial cancer originates in the endometrium, which is the lining of the uterus. Of all possible cancers of the female reproductive system, this one is the most commonly diagnosed. Rarely do physicians find endometrial cancer in women under the age of 40, and the most common age range is between age 50 and 69. Statistically speaking, survival rates are relatively high; about 83 percent of women who are diagnosed with endometrial cancer will survive it. There are more than a half million survivors of this type of cancer in the United States. Symptoms can include spotting or vaginal bleeding after menopause, extremely long periods, certain types of unusual discharge, and pain during sex. Obese women, women who have diabetes or polycystic ovary syndrome, and women who have infrequent periods are all at a higher risk for developing it.

Supportive Strategies for Preventing Endometrial Cancer

Annual gynecological exams. Women tend to be more diligent than men about yearly physical exams, perhaps because women are more informed about the importance of an annual gynecological exam. If, however, you're not vigilant about getting a checkup once a year, I implore you to put it on your calendar and not let a year go by without paying a visit to your gynecologist. Yearly exams, including a pelvic exam, are the first line of defense in preventing endometrial cancer.

Discuss HRT with your doctor. Just as with other types of cancer, certain methods of hormone replacement therapy (HRT) could be riskier than others, so be sure to discuss all the factors with your doctor before deciding on your HRT. Some studies show that estrogen alone can increase women's risk of endometrial cancer, though combining it with progesterone can lower this particular cancer risk. This is why I say to discuss it with your doctor, so you can come up with the plan that best fits you.

Act fast. If your periods change in any way, you have unusual discharge, or you experience bleeding during or after menopause, call your doctor right away. You may have something called endometrial hyperplasia, which has the ability to turn into endometrial cancer. Catch it early, and you could save your own life.

Ovarian Cancer

This deadly cancer can strike at any age, but older women are at a markedly higher risk. About 50 percent of diagnoses are in women over 60 years old. Sometimes ovarian cancer starts forming in the outside tissue of the ovary, whereas sometimes it originates in the actual egg-producing cells (germ cells). Another place it can start is in the ovarian cells responsible for producing hormones (estrogen and progesterone). While it is not the most common reproductive cancer for women, it is the deadliest, and all too often it isn't caught until it has progressed too far. There are some symptoms to watch for: swollen abdomen, persistent pain or tenderness in the pelvic region or lower back, gas that is resistant to treatment, and changes in bowel movements. Aside from age, other risk factors play a role. These include the presence of BRCA1 and BRCA2 (which also increase the risk of breast cancer), never giving birth, family history, and possibly the use of HRT.

Supportive Strategies for Preventing Ovarian Cancer

Consider oral contraception. There is pretty strong evidence that women who take birth control pills for at least five consecutive years have significantly lower chances of getting ovarian cancer. In fact, they may reduce their risk by 50 percent. It's worth discussing this option with your gynecologist.

Discuss genetic counseling. If you're very concerned about your risk because you have several family members who have been diagnosed with ovarian cancer, talk to your doctor about whether you should meet with a genetic counselor. This type of specialist can perform genetic testing. I advise you to do this only if you've really weighed the pros and cons of having this information. If you feel strongly that you'd want to have your ovaries removed if you found out you had a serious genetic risk of developing ovarian cancer, then have the testing done. If not, then this may not be the best route for you. I'm a believer that information is power, but others don't subscribe to that same philosophy when the information may be frightening.

Seek medical attention. If you suspect you have any signs of ovarian cancer, see your doctor. Don't delay, since the earlier it's caught, the better. Your doctor will perform testing such as a pelvic exam and ultrasound, and sometimes doctors will surgically remove some of the tissue for testing.

ANTI-CANCER CUISINE

Certain foods are basking in the limelight, thanks to their various anti-cancer properties. Get to your local grocery store or farmer's market to stock your fridge and fill your belly with the best and brightest in the army of anti-cancer fare.

Broccoli: This cruciferous veggie has glucosinolates that release certain enzymes when you chew it (especially when it's raw). Those enzymes can do some pretty amazing things like remove harmful substances and bacteria in your gut, which can add up to cancer protection.

Garlic: Various compounds in fresh garlic cloves could work some "magic" in your body. They can stop bacteria in their tracks, stop the formation of some substances known to cause cancer, boost repair of your DNA, and it's even possible that garlic can kill actual cancer cells. Buy fresh cloves, chop them up, and throw in tomato sauces, soups, steamed veggies, and other foods.

Carrots: These orange wonders of nature are loaded with beta-carotene, which could defend your body against invading cancer cells. Beta-carotene also packs an antioxidant wallop to certain viruses including HPV (human papilloma virus). Preserve the integrity of carrots' nutrients by steaming them whole, and cutting them up afterward.

Strawberries: Among other super-nutrients, strawberries offer ellagic acid, which can supercharge your body's ability to eradicate cancer cells. They also contain flavonoids, which are known to stop dangerous enzymes in their tracks before they have the potential to cause cancer. (Make room for other berries as well, including raspberries, blackberries, blueberries, and cranberries. Throw a bunch of different ones in a blender with some coconut water and sip on an anti-cancer smoothie!)

Swordfish: This yummy fish, along with other seafood delights such as sock-eye salmon and tuna (as well as cod liver oil, which you can take as a supplement), boasts some of the absolute highest levels of vitamin D of any foods found in nature. What does vitamin D have to do with preventing cancer? There's emerging research showing that it can actually slow the growth of cancer cells in your body. Go fish! (Or, at least eat some!)

Spinach: These leafy greens boast all kinds of anti-cancer deliciousness: lutein, zeaxanthin, and carotenoids are just a few. If you just can't stand the taste, throw handfuls of raw spinach into a blender along with a banana, coconut water, a little lemon juice, and a green apple. Trust me on this; it's delicious and you won't even know the spinach is in there!

Beans: Granted, eating pots of beans probably won't cure cancer, but they do contain saponins, phytic acid, and other compounds shown to offer protection to our bodies' cells against invading cancer cells. Plus, they're high in fiber. Soak dry beans first, and then cook them. Throw in a little fresh garlic for a one-two anti-cancer punch!

Grapes: These juicy round sensations (especially the red ones) have resveratrol, a type of phytochemical with anti-inflammatory properties. In one study, resveratrol hindered development of three different types of cancers. Munch on them plain, or chop them up and throw them in salads, include them in smoothies, or freeze them for a refreshing summertime snack.

Before you begin Cycle 3: Refine, take this quiz to find out how your reproductive system is faring. Then, after you complete the 17 Day Plan, take this quiz again to see how much you improved your score!

Women: Is Your Reproductive System on Its Way to 100 Happy, Healthy Years?

Answer each question honestly; give yourself the designated points for each answer. Add up your total and score yourself.

---

1. **Do you have irregular periods? (heavy bleeding, spotting in-between, periods longer than 7 days)**

    A. Yes ☐ 0 points

    B. No ☐ 4 points

    C. I don't have periods because I'm in menopause. ☐ 4 points

---

2. **If you're currently in menopause, have you had any random bleeding?**

    A. Yes ☐ 0 points

    B. No ☐ 4 points

    C. I'm not in menopause yet. ☐ 4 points

---

3. **Do you regularly experience pelvic pain or pressure?**

    A. Yes, and I haven't told my doctor. ☐ 0 points

    B. Yes, but I saw my doctor about it. ☐ 3 points

    C. No ☐ 4 points

---

4. **Do you constantly have a bloating or fullness sensation that nothing seems to help?**

    A. Yes, and I haven't told my doctor. ☐ 0 points

    B. Yes, but I saw my doctor about it. ☐ 3 points

    C. No ☐ 4 points

---

5. **In the last week, how many times did you have sex?**

    A. None ☐ 0 points

    B. One time ☐ 2 points

    C. Two or more times ☐ 4 points

---

6. **Have you gone for (or scheduled) your annual exam with your gynecologist?**

    A. No ☐ 0 points   B. Yes ☐ 4 points

7. **Do you have pain or discomfort during intercourse?**

   A. Yes ☐ 0 points   B. No ☐ 4 points

8. **How many days per week do you do cardio exercise?**

   A. None ☐ 0 points
   B. Once or twice ☐ 2 points
   C. Three or more times ☐ 4 points

9. **On an average week, what is your alcoholic intake?**

   A. Frequent (7+ drinks) ☐ 0 points
   B. Occasional (up to 6 drinks) ☐ 4 points

10. **Do you perform regular breast self-exams?**

    A. No ☐ 0 points   B. Yes ☐ 4 points

11. **Do you weigh yourself once per week?**

    A. No ☐ 0 points
    B. Yes, but I don't keep track. ☐ 1 point
    C. Yes, and I keep my weight in a healthy range. ☐ 4 points

12. **If you're nearing or in menopause, have you discussed HRT with your doctor?**

    A. I'm menopausal but I haven't met with my doctor. ☐ 0 points
    B. I'm menopausal and I have discussed an HRT plan. ☐ 4 points
    C. I'm not near menopause yet. ☐ 4 points

13. **If you have vaginal dryness, have you tried lubricants?**

    A. I have vaginal dryness, but I haven't tried lubricants. ☐ 0 points
    B. I have vaginal dryness and have tried lubricants. ☐ 4 points
    C. I don't have vaginal dryness. ☐ 4 points

14. **How often do you perform Kegel exercises?**

    A. Never ☐ 0 points
    B. Once a week ☐ 1 point
    C. Three or more times a week ☐ 2 points
    D. Every day ☐ 4 points

Scoring:

0–11: URGENT; see your gynecologist ASAP about any symptoms you're experiencing.

12–22: DANGEROUS; change your risky female reproductive system habits immediately.

23–33: MODERATELY RISKY; start doing more of my recommendations for improved reproductive system health.

34–44: AVERAGE; you have room for additional change.

45–56: EXCELLENT; stay on this positive course.

You probably got the point from this quiz (and the rest of the chapter) that if you're nearing menopause, you need to start weighing your options for coping with this stage of life. Your gynecologist is your biggest ally, teammate, and cheerleader in this new quest. If you're not happy with your doctor's recommendations, seek a second opinion.

Women, you have a tendency to put yourself last on your list of priorities. You are caretakers by nature, and the people in your life appreciate all that you do for them, even if they don't always say so. But those people also want you to be around for a very long time, and only *you* can take care of your health. Not that you need it, but I give you permission to put yourself *first* from this moment on. I want you to embrace getting older, not dread it. I want you to feel fabulous, because you, my dear, are a gift to be cherished!

CHAPTER 13

Macho, Macho Man

M en hate going to the doctor. I don't know if we equate illness with weakness, if we fear finding something wrong, or what. Maybe it's about money—that a visit might become exorbitant—or there could be a sense of embarrassment involved. I think we can be particularly bull-headed about our health, especially our sexual health.

Gentlemen, let me appeal to your logic. If you want all of your "parts" working well into your 100s, then you need to empower yourself right now, at whatever age you are, to protect the health of your reproductive system. And if the high cost of health care is your excuse, then let me assure you: If you neglect going to the doctor and getting regular checkups now, your long-term cost if something does go wrong will far exceed what you spend on those annual exams. That's because of a little thing we call "early detection." If you give your doctor a fighting chance to catch a problem early, you not only give yourself higher odds for survival, but you give your wallet a break, too.

But going to the doctor isn't just about looking for a tumor or signs of something serious. If you build and maintain a good relationship with your doctor, you'll feel more comfortable discussing issues like erectile dysfunction (it happens!) with him or her. And then you're more likely to get help solving it and getting relief. See how that works?

Look, as you get older, chances are that something will change with your reproductive system. In fact, there's a term for what happens to men as we age: It's called andropause. It refers to the steady decline of testosterone (an androgen), and symptoms can become apparent earlier than you may think—between ages 40 and 55. On average, male testosterone levels drop about 1 percent each year, beginning as early as age 30. This means that by the age of 70, you may have only half as much testosterone as you did in your 20s, or in some cases, even less than that. A drop in testosterone can bring about changes, whether subtle or drastic. Your libido may start fading, you may experience erectile dysfunction, or there may be physical changes you notice.

But I've got good news: You don't have to just accept these problems as they arise or live in fear of the day when they do. Remember, just because you're getting older doesn't mean you have to suffer with the "usual" indications of aging. There are ways around it, and no matter your current age, you can start right now to prevent a lot of these issues. In fact, my very first piece of advice is this: Use it or lose it. Sex, when physically safe and emotionally healthy, is good for your reproductive health. The more sex you have while you're young, the more likely you'll be able to have sex when you're much older. How's that for some doctor's orders?

Male Reproductive System 101

The male reproductive system is controlled by hormones, which we touched on in the endocrine system chapter. The hormones involved in male reproduction are follicle-stimulating hormone (FSH), testosterone (T), and luteinizing hormone (LH). Both your FSH and LH are secreted by the pituitary gland, located in the brain. They then travel down to the testes, where they connect with receptors, and the LH causes testosterone to be produced while the FSH causes sperm to be produced. Testosterone plays a big role in your innately male attributes: facial hair, low voice, muscles, libido, and so on. But testosterone levels wane as men age, which can cause changes to the male reproductive system on the whole.

The prostate, which we will also discuss in the urinary chapter because it can have an impact on urinary functioning, is actually part of the male reproductive system. Its role is to provide fluids in which the sperm can travel and remain healthy. The prostate is quite susceptible to the five factors of aging, particularly inflammation. Many men experience discomfort or health issues with their prostate as they get older, but we'll discuss preventative measures in this chapter.

The penis is the organ by which semen, and thus sperm, is expelled. The penis is obviously a key topic within male sexuality, and just like the prostate, its functioning can be affected by aging. Erectile dysfunction is an extremely common issue among the aging male population, but the fantastic news is that we can both prevent it and reverse it.

Now let's tackle some of the age-related issues we guys may experience and what we can do about them!

How the Male Reproductive System Ages

As you know, women go through menopause when they are no longer fertile. Men remain fertile longer than women do, but they do experience a decrease in male sex hormones. That period of time and the symptoms that come with it is sometimes referred to as andropause.

Andropause is nothing like menopause. It's gradual and may have less impact on men than menopause typically does on women. Along with the drop in testosterone, the testicles themselves can shrink slightly, sex drive can drop, sperm count can decrease, breast tissue and fat can increase, bones can become more fragile, and sleep can become difficult. Furthermore, a man in andropause may experience problems with achieving or maintaining erections. Sperm production can also slow down, while the internal tubes that transfer sperm can stiffen and lose some of their elasticity. The prostate can get larger over time, because the tissue becomes like scar tissue, and it can also become inflamed. Those issues can interfere with both urination and ejaculation. Other prostate changes as we age can lead to frequent urinary tract infections. One more thing: The risk of prostate cancer increases with age.

Now, on to how to stop or avoid all that!

A SUPPLEMENT THAT SUPPORTS MALE REPRODUCTIVE SYSTEM

● **Saw Palmetto**—taken as directed

Why: If you do a little research, you'll find that the jury is still out on whether this herb actually has a positive effect on prostate symptoms. Still, I think it's worth a try. It might actually improve the overall health of your prostate and help prevent enlarged prostate. I'm not saying it's a miracle cure, but many of my patients swear by it. Make sure you're choosing a high-quality saw palmetto supplement. The regulations aren't super strict on herbal supplements, so pick a reputable company to get the most effective supplement.

The Number-One Strategy: Stop Inflammation

Inflammation, your body's wildfire, has harmful effects on all of your body's systems, but there's an intriguing connection between inflammation and testosterone. It turns out that a normal amount of testosterone in the body can actually fight inflammation. As we've discussed, obesity and belly fat can be a main cause of inflammation in the body, and they can also contribute to lower production of testosterone. If you have a high amount of CRP (C-reactive protein), a marker for inflammation, you're at a huge risk for erectile dysfunction (not to mention a host of other serious health problems and symptoms). High CRP also means a higher risk of prostate cancer. Are you convinced? We want to stop the inflammation in your body so that all your male parts can function at their peak!

The Anti-Aging Essentials and Your Reproductive System

#1: Movement. Anytime one of my patients is experiencing erectile dysfunction (ED), my very first question is, "Are you exercising regularly?" And the moment I detect hesitation, all I can say is, "Get moving!" The very first line of defense against ED is to spend at least 30 minutes a day increasing your heart rate through movement. I don't care if you're swimming, jogging, climbing stairs, or doing jumping jacks—any of it will help prevent and reverse ED. Get yourself a heart monitor and get to your target heart rate every day. Not sure what your target heart rate should be during a workout? Subtract your age from 220. That number is your maximum heart rate. Your *cardio zone* is 60 to 80 percent of your maximum heart rate. Simple! This will work wonders on your sex life, as well as the rest of your life.

#2: Maintain a healthy weight. Studies show that the more overweight you are, the more likely you are to have a low sperm count or even produce no sperm at all. One theory on why this happens is that testosterone may get converted to estrogen in the excess fatty tissue. Researchers also

speculate that the excess fat around the lower abdominal area could cause the scrotum to overheat, thus affecting sperm production.

If you're overweight, your first order of business is to get into a healthy weight range. This step alone will lower your overall inflammation. Other factors that play roles in promoting inflammation are too much alcohol, smoking, certain foods (some that will surprise you), eating the wrong fats, too much table salt, and lots more. I'll incorporate methods for reducing inflammation in the supportive strategies below.

#3: Stay hydrated. Even slight dehydration can negatively impact sperm production. Just by drinking six to eight 8-ounce glasses of water daily, you are contributing to healthy amounts of sperm production and semen volume.

#4: Avoid smoking. Tobacco use also lowers sperm count, damages the sperm, and thus decreases overall fertility. There's a certain protein that sperm carry and researchers discovered that smokers' sperm don't carry as much of it, making them susceptible to DNA damage. Smoking also increases free radical production within semen.

#5: Supplements. Continue taking your multivitamin and any other supplements mentioned in other chapters that the multi doesn't cover, but consider adding saw palmetto, especially if you're concerned about prostate health.

Age-Related Male Reproductive Issues

Low Testosterone (Low T)

First, go get your testosterone levels checked if you haven't already done so. The normal range is wide—between 200 and 800 ng/dL. Every guy has a different "healthy" measurement of testosterone, so I actually think it's a smart idea to get your levels checked at a young age to get a baseline. That way, you'll know if you're really out of whack later on. Regardless, get tested ASAP so you know what you're working with.

Symptoms of low testosterone include decreased interest in sex (low libido), trouble with erections, depression, overall feeling of fatigue, weight gain (particularly fat gain), increased breast tissue, and insomnia. In the long run, it can even make your bones more brittle. In 2010, a British study done on male heart disease patients elicited surprising results. The men in the group who also had low testosterone had a greater chance of dying than the men with normal testosterone levels. The media grabbed on to these results and ran with lots of stories about how low T can kill you. Perhaps the data were sensationalized, but I think it's worth taking into account that low T really doesn't do you any favors at all. It's pretty astounding how important that hormone is to your overall health, isn't it? Plus, it doesn't get low just due to aging. There are other possible causes, including testicular injury or cancer, endocrine disorders, certain types of infection, HIV, type 2 diabetes, and obesity.

There's actually some research showing that one in four men who are 30 years old or older fall in the category of low T. Those numbers may be even higher, because many men don't seek treatment. Like I said, some guys just hate going to the doctor, but in the case of low T, many men also don't know what signs to look for. So aside from low libido, consider seeing your physician if you have any of the following: fatigue, depression, moodiness, changes in cholesterol levels, decreases in genital sensitivity, weight gain, decrease in muscle and testicle size, and hair loss.

Supportive Strategies for Low Testosterone

The main strategy for boosting testosterone levels is through testosterone replacement (naturally and synthetically). This isn't as drastic as it may sound—it's just a treatment to boost a deficiency in testosterone. If you've been diagnosed with low testosterone, this is a great way to start feeling like yourself again. It can boost libido and energy, help muscles grow, fight depression, and so on. There are various methods for replacing your testosterone. One option is a patch that you apply to your skin each day, which works to slowly release testosterone into your body the same way a nicotine patch releases nicotine. There are also gels that your skin absorbs, a patch that goes in your mouth, and pills, as well as a number of other options. It seems the least invasive methods could be the most effective, and they carry the fewest risks. Your doctor will work with you to decide on the best form for you. But seriously, guys, don't delay. Low T is nothing to be embarrassed about and it's something that you can so easily reverse.

Erectile Dysfunction (ED)

This is such a touchy subject because if we can't perform sexually, we feel like less of a man. It's just how we're wired. But ED is not inevitable as we age, and if you do have it, there's nothing to be embarrassed about. I'm on a mission to get men to put the shame aside and realize that so many others, 30 million American men in fact, go through it. ED can be brought on by lack of movement (exercise), stress, low testosterone or other reproductive system issues, obesity, heart disease, certain medications, tobacco use, high blood pressure, high cholesterol, diabetes, or psychological matters. Let's define ED, though, because if you just have the occasional problem achieving an erection (say, after a celebration at the local bar), you probably don't fall in this category. Erectile dysfunction, requiring treatment, is usually defined by the inability to get an erection or maintain it more than 50 percent of the time.

Supportive Strategies for Erectile Dysfunction

Eat what's good for your heart. Food that is healthy for your heart is also healthy for your reproductive system. Essentially, fatty, greasy foods negatively impact circulation, and since erections are about blood flow, you can imagine how poor circulation can lead to erectile dysfunction. So load up your diet with fruits, vegetables, whole grains, lean proteins, and healthy fats instead of burgers and fries. When it comes time to perform, you'll be glad you did!

Stress less. We know stress can get our hormones out of whack, and one of those hormones that is sensitive to stress is adrenaline. Too much adrenaline can cause the blood vessels to contract, which can inhibit an erection. If you're experiencing ED for the first time and you also have other new stress going on in your life, I can guarantee there is a connection. Figure out a healthy method that helps you relax (meditation, deep breathing, stretching, journaling, etc.) and do that daily.

Consider a prescription. If exercise and focusing on stressing less don't solve your problem down there, you should consider talking to your doctor about erectile dysfunction medications. They can have side effects (including headache, flushing, changes in vision, back pain, and stomach problems) and they aren't for everyone (especially if you've had arrhythmia or a recent heart attack), but for many men, these drugs can really help.

Enlarged Prostate

Ninety percent of men in their 70s and 80s have an enlarged prostate. It's often referred to as BPH, benign prostatic hyperplasia. Here's the good news: It doesn't increase your risk of getting prostate cancer later on. And the bad news: It can interfere with your urination and cause various urinary tract problems. Some signs of BPH are a weak urine stream, frequent need to urinate, and straining during urination. While we're not 100 percent certain of the causes of BPH, it could have to do with changes in male hormones.

Supportive Strategies for Enlarged Prostate

Reduce certain OTC drugs. If you're taking decongestants or antihistamines for your allergies or cold symptoms and are also having symptoms of an enlarged prostate, you should taper off these drugs with the help of your physician. That's because they are known to tighten the muscles near your urethra, making urination more difficult.

No nighttime sipping. Try to quit drinking any fluids in the two to three hours leading up to bedtime. This will help reduce the middle-of-the-night trips to the bathroom that an enlarged prostate can often cause.

Slow down the booze and coffee. Both caffeine and alcohol generally stimulate your bladder, thus they can make urination symptoms associated with enlarged prostate worse.

Consider meds. Your doctor can prescribe medications if your enlarged prostate is causing problems for you. Alpha blockers, among other types of drugs, might relieve your symptoms.

Discuss surgery with your doctor. If you have an enlarged prostate and it's interfering with your life, there are surgical options that can help.

I know it's frightening to think about having any part of your reproductive system surgically removed, but trust me when I say this surgery isn't nearly as big a deal as you might imagine. There are minimally invasive options available. If you're suffering, it's worth discussing this with your doctor.

Prostatitis

Protastitis is an inflamed or swollen prostate. There are different types, some of which are caused by a bacterial infection. This condition doesn't always have symptoms, but when it does, they include abdominal, groin, and lower back pain; pain during orgasm; flu symptoms; urination troubles, and more. Important: Prostatitis is different from an enlarged prostate. It actually occurs more often in younger or middle-aged patients. You can get it from unprotected sex, dehydration, infection, and even stress.

Supportive Strategies for Prostatitis

Wash well. You have to have good hygiene, fellas. Since some types of prostatitis are caused by bacteria, you can prevent that by properly cleaning your penis. If you're uncircumcised, be sure to pull back the foreskin in the shower and wash with soap and water, but always rinse well. Take a shower as soon as possible after a workout or sex so that bacteria don't have a chance to grow. And drink enough water to flush out your urethra.

Discuss meds with your doctor. If you've been diagnosed already, medications such as antibiotics might be recommended. But discuss this with your doctor. Other meds your doctor could suggest are alpha blockers, pain relievers, and anti-inflammatory meds.

Avoid sitting for long periods. If you have a job where you're sitting all day or your exercise of choice is long-distance bike riding, your prostate health may be at risk. Try mixing up your cardiovascular exercise and be sure to stand up and walk around at least once every hour at work.

Testicular Cancer

This form of cancer isn't necessarily related to aging, but it's worth bringing it up in this chapter because I want all of you guys to be cognizant of it, and to understand how to conduct self-exams. Just because it's rarer than other forms of cancer doesn't mean we should bury our heads in the sand! It's also very treatable, which is great news. The symptoms include a feeling of heaviness in the scrotum, a swollen testicle or a lump you can feel, achiness in the groin or lower abdominal area or testicular pain, and enlargement or tenderness in breast tissue. The majority of testicular cancer diagnoses are in men who have no family history of it, although if someone in your family had it, you are at a slightly higher risk.

Supportive Strategies for Testicular Cancer

If you suspect you have testicular cancer, I advise you to immediately see your doctor. Do not wait. Your physician can perform an ultrasound and do blood tests, and if you're diagnosed with cancer, will work together with you to create a treatment plan, which will depend upon the stage at which it was diagnosed. In some cases, doctors recommend having the testicle and surrounding lymph nodes surgically removed, followed by radiation or chemotherapy to destroy any remaining cancer cells.

As I said, this is a very survivable cancer, but early detection is the key. There's not really much you can do to prevent this type of cancer, but self-exams and routine screenings are your strategy.

TESTICULAR CANCER SELF-EXAM

It might be easiest to perform this self-exam immediately following a shower or when you're warm, so the scrotum is loose and relaxed. First, inspect your scrotum in the mirror. You're looking for swelling. Next, roll one testicle at a time around between your fingers and thumbs. Do they feel normal? Or is one suddenly larger than it was or swollen? Do you feel any lumps or bumps? Closely inspect all aspects of the testicles and scrotum. If everything is normal, repeat in 30 days. If you detect any changes, see your doctor ASAP.

Before you begin Cycle 3: Refine, take this quiz to find out how your reproductive system is faring. Then, after you complete the 17 Day Plan, take this quiz again to see how much you improved your score!

Men: Is Your Reproductive System on Its Way to 100 Happy, Healthy Years?

1. **In the past week, have you reached your target heart rate for 30 minutes on at least five days?**

    A. No ☐ 0 points   B. Yes ☐ 4 points

2. **Do you have trouble achieving or maintaining an erection 50 percent or more of the time?**

    A. Yes ☐ 0 points   B. No ☐ 4 points

3. **How much caffeine do you consume?**

    A. Three or more servings per day ☐ 0 points
    B. One serving per day or less ☐ 3 points
    C. I don't consume caffeine regularly. ☐ 4 points

4. **Have you had your testosterone level checked?**

    A. No ☐ 0 points   B. Yes ☐ 4 points

5. **Do you have a family history of prostate cancer?**

    A. Yes ☐ 0 points   B. No ☐ 4 points

6. **In the last week, how many times did you have sex?**

    A. None ☐ 0 points
    B. One time ☐ 2 points
    C. Two or more times ☐ 4 points

7. **If you've had ED symptoms, did you discuss them with your doctor?**

    A. I've had symptoms, but haven't talked to a doctor. ☐ 0 points
    B. I've had symptoms and discussed them with a doctor. ☐ 3 points
    C. I've never had symptoms. ☐ 4 points

8. **Do you maintain excellent penile hygiene?**

   A. No ☐ 0 points   B. Yes ☐ 4 points

9. **Do you perform regular testicular self-exams?**

   A. No ☐ 0 points   B. Yes ☐ 4 points

10. **In the last week, how often has your stress level been high?**

   A. Often—consistently at a 5+ on scale of 1 to 10 ☐ 0 points
   B. Sometimes—two to three days per week, I'm at a 5+ on scale of 1 to 10. ☐ 1 points
   C. Rarely—only at a 5 on scale of 1 to 10 once. ☐ 3 points
   D. No—I almost never feel stressed. ☐ 4 points

11. **Is your testosterone level considered normal?**

   A. I don't know. ☐ 0 points
   B. It's low, but I'm not undergoing treatment. ☐ 1 point
   C. It's low, and I'm getting treatment. ☐ 3 points
   D. Yes, my testosterone is normal. ☐ 4 points

12. **Do you take saw palmetto?**

   A. No ☐ 0 points   B. Yes ☐ 4 points

13. **Is your diet high in animal proteins but low in veggies?**

   A. Yes ☐ 0 points   B. No ☐ 4 points

14. **Have you gone for an annual checkup with your doctor or urologist?**

   A. No ☐ 0 points   B. Yes ☐ 4 points

Scoring:

0–11: URGENT; see your doctor ASAP about any symptoms you may be experiencing.

12–22: DANGEROUS; immediately change your risky reproductive system habits.

23–33: MODERATELY RISKY; include more of my suggestions in your routine to improve the functioning of your reproductive system.

34–44: AVERAGE; you have room for additional change.

45–56: EXCELLENT; stay on this positive course.

How did you score? In the Cycle 3 17 Day Plan, you'll find daily assignments designed to improve the health of your reproductive system. After the 17 days, take the quiz again to see your improvements. I hope you notice change for the better in the bedroom (or somewhere more creative), too!

Guys, your sexual health can be an excellent indicator of your overall health. And while keeping your sex life healthy is probably a priority for you, it's good to keep in mind that some sexual problems are early signs of more serious illnesses. In other words, you've got to take your reproductive health seriously. Don't ignore sexual symptoms down there or assume they'll work themselves out. If you talk it out with your doctor, you might find that a simple tune-up will get you back in the race. But if you delay, you could actually miss a chance at early diagnosis and treatment for something else.

CHAPTER 14

Keep Your Stream Steady

L et's talk about something that some of us have to admit we struggle with: urinary problems. It can be scary to discover that going to the bathroom is no longer the straightforward, pain-free bodily activity it once was for you, and that's probably why a lot of people keep the issue to themselves. Urinary issues can also feel embarrassing, even shameful. But did you know that literally millions of people are suffering in silence over problems "down there"? Breaking the silence is the first step toward getting help for these demoralizing, often debilitating, but treatable conditions.

As you get older, it's normal to urinate more frequently because your bladder loses some of its capacity. It becomes increasingly inflexible, and it contracts, making it harder to hold as much. While the urge to pee more often is a normal part of getting older, urinary incontinence (UI), which is the sudden, uncontrollable need to urinate, is not. Urinary incontinence strikes approximately 200 million adults around the world every day. But here's the stat that really bothers me: One out of 10 folks over 65 years old suffers with UI. As you might imagine, UI can significantly affect your quality of life. It really doesn't have to be that way, and I am determined to help you avoid having to deal with this potentially devastating ailment as you get older.

In order to prevent or control incontinence and other urine-related problems, you must first understand the basics of the urinary system. Here we go.

Urinary System 101

The organs involved in your urinary system are your bladder, ureters, kidneys, sphincter muscles, and urethra. They all work together to generate and store urine. Your bladder, a balloon-shaped organ, is your urine storage unit. Urine is housed there until you're ready to release it through the urethra and out of your body.

Other organs in your body, such as your skin, intestines, and lungs, also excrete waste, and they rely on your urinary system to help with this process. Think of this system as your body's trash chute: All the other systems we've talked about so far throw their excess waste into it.

On average, we pee about a quart and a half of urine each day. Urine is a combination of urea (a by-product of the protein you've consumed) and other waste by-products from around your body. Sitting near the middle of your back, just below your rib cage, are your kidneys. They extract urea out of your blood through tiny filtering units called nephrons. Once through the kidneys, urine travels down the ureters into the bladder. Circular muscles called sphincters help keep urine from leaking by tightening down around the bladder opening into the urethra.

Once there's enough urine inside your bladder, you'll begin feeling the need to head to the bathroom. As the bladder continues to fill, the urge to urinate gets stronger until you empty it. During urination, the bladder muscle contracts, the sphincter muscles let go of their grip, and pelvic muscles relax so that urine can exit the bladder, travel through the urethra, and flow out of your body. If all goes well, this entire process occurs on your terms, in the bathroom and not before you can make it to the toilet.

SUPPLEMENTS THAT SUPPORT THE URINARY SYSTEM

- **Vitamin C:** 1,000 mg daily
- **Antioxidant multivitamin:** Take as directed on the bottle.
- **Calcium:** 1,000 mg daily
- **Magnesium:** 400 mg daily

Why: Vitamin C can halt the growth of "bad" bacteria in your urine. Take a multiple antioxidant supplement. Alternatively (or better yet—additionally!), eat lots of orange and yellow veggies and fruit—they're loaded to the max with beta-carotene. Together, calcium and magnesium help improve control of the muscles used in urination.

Dr. Mike's Cranberry Mocktail

I'm a believer in supplementing your diet with cranberry because of the positive effects its hippuric acid has on your urinary tract. No, it is not a cure for a urinary tract infection, so if you're experiencing symptoms, go to your doctor and take antibiotics if they're prescribed for you. It is, however, a terrific way to prevent "bad" bacteria from accumulating in your urethra, where they can thrive and cause infection.

Sure, you can take a cranberry pill supplement and enjoy the benefits. But if you're in the mood for a "mocktail," here's a fun recipe. Pucker up; it can be tart!

Two 1-ounce shots of unsweetened cranberry juice
Juice of ½ orange
1 teaspoon agave nectar or honey (or any natural
    sweetener)
½ cup seltzer or club soda
Ice
Optional: Fresh mint leaves

Combine the ingredients in a martini shaker, gently shake or stir, then strain through the ice and pour into a martini glass. Garnish with mint leaves and enjoy. Cheers to your urinary health!

How the Urinary System Ages

As you get older, your kidneys change structurally. They don't perform their waste removal job as effectively. Also, the muscles in your ureters, bladder, and urethra tend to lose some of their strength. A loss of strength in these muscles can cause incontinence. Many older people also experience an increase in various urinary infections because the bladder muscles don't tighten enough to empty their bladder completely.

Doctors can detect urinary problems through various tests. Urinalysis, for example, is a test that looks at urine to detect protein, signs of infection, or other abnormal substances. I'm sure you've done this routine before: At your doctor's office, you urinate into a little cup and leave the sample to be closely studied. If you're having trouble with the muscles or nerves of your urinary system and pelvis, your doctor may want to do a "urodynamic test." This test evaluates how well your urine is stored and whether or not it exits from your bladder normally. There are other bladder tests that use dyes and x-ray to see whether the bladder fills and empties normally.

Problems of the urinary system range in severity from mild to life-threatening:

Urinary incontinence. Those who suffer from a lack of bladder control may leak a little or have no ability at all to gauge when they need to urinate. Leakage can occur when you laugh, cough, bend over, or lift something, or even while walking. Different issues can lead to incontinence, including childbirth, stress, and just aging. There are many ways to treat it successfully. Your doctor may recommend treatments from simple exercises to surgery. Women suffer from urinary incontinence more often than men. Fortunately, there are easy ways to prevent and manage this very annoying problem, including some simple bladder-training exercises.

Urinary tract infections (UTIs). These sometimes painful infections are caused by the presence of "bad" bacteria inside your urinary tract. Women get UTIs more often than men. Antibiotics will typically clear up UTIs in no time. Drinking lots of fluids also helps by flushing out the bacteria. The type of UTI depends on its location. For example, cystitis refers to a bladder infection, while pyelonephritis is a kidney infection. This type of UTI can seriously damage your kidneys if not promptly treated. I've designed a special "mocktail" (see 201) using cranberry juice that you'll love.

Interstitial cystitis (IC). This is a chronic, inflammatory bladder disorder affecting the walls of your bladder. Ultimately, it can cause the bladder to become less elastic and can lower its capacity. Other symptoms are bleeding and, in rare cases, ulcers in the bladder lining.

Interstitial cystitis is a challenging condition to treat. It responds well to various drugs, including antidepressants, which relax the bladder; antihistamines, which control inflammation and reduce the urgency to pee;

and painkillers, which relieve the pain. Giving up caffeine-loaded beverages such as coffee and sodas is important too, since caffeine irritates the bladder and causes discomfort in people who suffer from this condition. It's best, though, to try to prevent interstitial cystitis from happening in the first place. That can be done with bladder training, stress management techniques, adequate hydration, and supplements that control inflammation and oxidative stress.

Kidney stones. Not that any of these malfunctions are a barrel of laughs, but kidney stones can be particularly miserable. They're tiny things called calculi that develop inside the urinary system, not necessarily just the kidneys. Certain factors put you at higher risk for developing these stones: obesity, diets excessively high in protein, diets high in sodium, dehydration, family history, and frequent urinary tract infections. The goal of treatment is to eliminate the stones completely, prevent infection, and prevent them from forming again. Both nonsurgical and surgical treatments are used. Men suffer from kidney stones more often than women. Protecting your kidneys is much like protecting any other organ in your body: through weight control, proper nutrition, and adequate hydration.

Nocturia. This is when you have to wake up from sleep in order to urinate. If you've ever been pregnant, you're familiar with having to get out of bed to pee. But if you're not pregnant, it's worth discussing with your doctor because it can be a symptom of chronic urinary tract infections, cystitis, or benign prostatic hyperplasia (which I'll explain below). One of the simplest ways to control this condition is to not drink any liquids three hours prior to bedtime.

Proteinuria. This is when you have abnormal amounts of protein in your urine, which may be a sign that your kidneys are not working properly. Proteinuria may be caused by inflammation, and contributing factors may include diabetes, heart disease, high blood pressure, and kidney disease. The best way to find out if you have this condition is with a simple urine test; if you do, follow-up testing will help detect the cause.

To prevent and manage this condition, ease up on your salt intake. Salt decreases the amount of water in your body. Lower your blood pressure. Proteinuria is often found in combination with high blood pressure because high blood pressure weakens capillaries in the kidneys. Cut back on the amount of protein you eat; simply eat smaller portions of protein at each meal, or emphasize more plant proteins, such as beans and legumes. Also, keep tabs on your blood sugar levels if they tend to be high, because there's a direct link between diabetes and proteinuria.

Renal (kidney) failure. This is the result of your kidneys not adequately removing waste products from your blood. There are two kinds of kidney failure: acute renal failure (ARF) and chronic renal failure (CRF). ARF comes on suddenly, and it's usually due to some kind of physical trauma or blood loss, or even poisoning or drugs. ARF is quite serious and may permanently impair your kidneys. Unlike ARF, with CRF there is a slow decline in the function of your kidneys. It may cause permanent kidney failure, or end-stage renal disease (ESRD).

In general, keeping kidneys healthy means following a low-sodium diet, controlling blood sugar, drinking ample amounts of water, and eating lots of fruits and vegetables (this helps you to better excrete kidney-stone-inhibiting citrate into your urine).

MY TOP LOW-SODIUM FOODS

Too much sodium causes water retention, contributes to high blood pressure, and increases your risk of urinary problems. The American Heart Association and other experts recommend we limit our dietary sodium to 2,300 milligrams (about one teaspoon of table salt) a day for healthy adults up to age 50 and 1,500 milligrams a day for people age 51 or older, African-Americans, and those with high blood pressure, diabetes, or kidney disease. But many of us consume five or more teaspoons of sodium daily. To help you reduce the sodium in your diet, here's my personal list of the best low-sodium foods.

Fresh vegetables: Generally, canned veggies are loaded with sodium, so stick to fresh produce whenever possible.

Fresh fruits: Similarly to vegetables, fresh fruit is lower in sodium than if packaged or canned.

Nuts: Unsalted and natural will give you the crunch, without the sodium.

Low-sodium varieties of your favorite foods: Fortunately, food makers are catering to the low-sodium crowd by reducing added salt in foods. Search out low-salt versions of your favorite soups, condiments, crackers, chips, and popcorns. I recommend avoiding products containing more than 200 milligrams of sodium per serving. Also, check the ingredients list for hidden sodium sources, such as baking soda/powder, monosodium glutamate, and any substance containing the word "sodium."

Salmon: This fish is low in sodium. No need to add any, either; just sprinkle it with healthy, flavor-friendly herbs and spices.

Whole-grain cereals: These include oatmeal, cream of wheat, and cream of rice, but be sure to prepare them without adding salt.

DECODE LOW-SODIUM LABELING

Get familiar with these labels when shopping for low-sodium foods:

Sodium/salt-free: Less than 5 milligrams of sodium per serving
Very low sodium: 35 milligrams of sodium or less per serving
Low sodium: 140 milligrams of sodium or less per serving
Reduced sodium: Product has at least 25 percent less sodium than regular version.
Light: Product has at least 50 percent less sodium than regular version.

Age-Related Urinary Problems Pertaining Only to Men

Prostatitis. Often with prostatitis, you feel an urge to urinate a lot more often, and it can hurt when you urinate. You might also have pain in your lower back and genital area. Prostatitis is simply the result of an inflamed prostate gland and often can be treated with antibiotics. However, if you're experiencing symptoms, don't make assumptions. Always see your doctor when symptoms appear. If you're practicing my anti-inflammation and immune-boosting strategies, you're going a long way toward preventing prostatitis.

Benign prostatic hyperplasia (BPH). This is the technical name for an enlarged prostate. While it's actually part of your reproductive system, the prostate is positioned near the bladder and urethra, so it makes sense that its enlargement would have a negative effect on your urinary system.

Usually, this disorder blocks urine flow by squeezing the urethra, making it hard to pee—patients will often have to strain in order to start urinating. Other problems, including the urge to pee more often, can occur. Many men over the age of 60 experience some BPH. It can be successfully treated by removing part of the prostate using laser, microwave, or traditional surgery, making it possible to urinate normally again. Don't worry; usually, neither libido nor sexual ability is affected. I discuss this topic in more depth in the male reproductive system chapter.

Also, a lot of men who have BPH benefit from taking saw palmetto supplements. Available in health food stores, saw palmetto is an herb that helps shrink the prostate. It may also increase your sex drive!

Prostate cancer. Prostate cancer is at the top of the list of cancer deaths in men (approximately 30,000 annually), second only to lung cancer. One out of six men have risk factors for prostate cancer. It is more commonly found in older men, but younger guys are not exempt. No one has yet pinpointed causes for prostate cancer, but research points to family history and a high-fat diet. If you're over the age of 40, consult your doctor regarding your prostate health. You should discuss family history, the possibility of having a PSA (prostate specific antigen) test, and most importantly, having a digital rectal exam. If you are diagnosed, there are multiple variations of treatment regimens depending on your diagnosis and recommendations from your physician. Some treatment options include watchful waiting, active surveillance, hormone therapy, chemotherapy, and partial or radical surgery.

As for prevention, studies show that consuming enough lycopene, an antioxidant found in tomatoes, is key. You can pop lycopene supplements, but the best preventive action comes from cooked tomato products, such as tomato paste and sauce. Tomato processing makes lycopene more absorbable in your body. Another prevention tip: Cut back on animal fat, found in fatty meats and butter. The more animal fat you eat, the greater your prostate cancer risk.

Anti-Aging Essentials and Your Urinary System

#1: Movement. Exercise can decrease stagnation of urine within the bladder, thus decreasing your risk of getting a urinary tract infection.

#2: Maintain a healthy weight. Adjusting your diet and lifestyle to keep your weight in a healthy range is a big part of helping your urinary tract function properly. Obese people run a higher risk of getting both kidney stones and urinary tract infections. Researchers speculate that obesity causes an imbalance of certain chemicals in the blood, thus increasing the likelihood of developing stones. Improve your urinary health today simply by choosing one "guilty pleasure" food you indulge in often and giving it a healthy makeover. For instance, are you a pizza lover? Try ordering your next pie with a thin crust, extra sauce, no cheese, and at least four veggie toppings. Yum!

#3: Stay hydrated. Keep drinking water! Some people with urinary problems may restrict the amount of water they're drinking, thinking it will help them lower the number of accidents they have by urinating less frequently. But, as we age, we are more likely to suffer deleterious effects of dehydration, in a shorter amount of time. Furthermore, drinking plenty of water every day helps keep your urinary tract flushed out (no pun intended). Keep drinking my recommended six to eight cups of water daily.

#4: Avoid smoking. Sure, you already know that smoking can lead to cancer of the lungs. But it turns out that even the urinary system is not exempt from the health effects of smoking. A group of researchers analyzed dozens of studies on smokers and concluded that, when compared to nonsmokers, smokers are three times more likely to get cancer of the urinary tract. I'm not trying to scare you; I just want you to draw the connection between smoking and literally every system in your body.

#5: Supplements. Refer to the supplement section in this chapter to find out which vitamins and nutrients can support your urinary system.

The Number-One Strategy: Boost Immunity

Heredity and aging may play a role, but nobody should sit back and wait for the onset of illness in their urinary system. A huge factor in most of these problems has to do with immunity. If you can keep your immune system strong and healthy, you'll go a long way toward keeping your urinary system in peak condition. There are easy ways to do this, measures that we all should be taking but many of us aren't. For example, drinking cranberry juice and eating blueberries are two of the best things you can do, starting right now. These berries contain substances that keep bacteria from sticking to the tissues of the bladder and causing an infection. Another simple nutritional tip is to include foods high in potassium in your diet, especially if you are prone to kidney stones. Potassium can help prevent the formation of stones because it attaches to calcium deposits, so get your fill of citrus fruits, bananas, coconut water, dried apricots, yogurt, tomatoes, potatoes, and most green vegetables.

URINE COLORS DECODED

When you go to the bathroom, it's a good idea to take note of the color of your urine. Here's a list of colors to look for and what they can tell you about your health.

Faint yellow: This is considered a normal urine color. Urine gets lighter in color the more water you drink.

Dark yellow: Can indicate dehydration. Drink more water and see if it changes.

Red or pink: Can be caused by eating beets or other red foods or dyes, certain medications such as antibiotics, laxatives, and some meds that ease urinary pain. It can also mean there is blood in your urine. This sometimes occurs in distance runners. But if those things don't apply, blood in urine can indicate something much more serious, ranging from urinary tract infections to kidney stones, cysts or tumors, enlarged prostate, and more, so see your doctor ASAP.

Dark brown: Certain foods such as fava beans and rhubarb can cause this, as well as several medications. Some kidney and liver disorders sometimes turn urine this color too. See your doctor, especially if this persists.

Orange: Medications such as antibiotics, laxatives, and some chemotherapy drugs can cause urine to turn orange. Medical conditions involving the liver or bile duct can also cause this.

Cloudy or murky: Can indicate kidney stones or urinary tract infection. See your doctor.

Limit alcohol and caffeine. These beverages can worsen urinary symptoms, particularly incontinence (since both make you pee more often).

Train your bladder through exercise. Just like any muscle, your bladder needs to be exercised. The more you're able to exercise your urinary muscles, the lower your risk for urinary incontinence later on. Plus, this strength routine can improve UI symptoms if you already suffer from them. They're called Kegel exercises. Yes, this exercise has benefits for *both* women and men! Here's what to do: First, to familiarize yourself with the pelvic muscles, try to stop the flow of urination halfway through. When it stops, you know you've just used the muscles we're targeting. Don't squeeze your legs, buttocks, or abdominal muscles, though. You want to isolate the pelvic floor. You'll feel a pulling sensation when you flex these muscles. Now you're ready to give them a workout! You can do this anywhere, anytime—no one will even know. Simply contract the muscles for five seconds, then release for five seconds. Repeat the process until you've done 10 reps.

Make toilet appointments. Here's something else that you can do on your own to control urinary incontinence: Schedule specific times for visiting the restroom, preferably every two to four hours. This way, you run less of a risk of "holding it" longer than you should.

Limit foods that irritate your bladder. If you're currently experiencing urinary pain or other symptoms, you should limit highly acidic foods like citrus fruits, sugary foods like honey or sweet desserts, and foods that contain caffeine, including chocolate and sodas. If you're not currently having symptoms, however, citrus fruits can be beneficial in reducing the risk of stone formation.

Not to pick on caffeine, but it is a bladder irritant. It stimulates spasms in sensitive nerves and bladder muscles, plus acts as a diuretic (which means more trips to the bathroom). If you've been having urinary problems, I'd suggest cutting back on caffeine (no more than one cup of coffee a day) or cutting it out altogether.

Soon you'll be starting Refine Cycle 3 to improve your urinary and reproductive systems. Before you begin that plan, take this quiz to determine your overall urinary health. Then, after you complete the 17 days, take this quiz again to see how much you improved your score!

Is Your Urinary System on Its Way to 100 Happy, Healthy Years?

Answer each question honestly; give yourself the designated points for each answer. Add up your total and score yourself.

1. **Recently, have you detected blood in your urine?**

   A. Yes ☐ 0 points   B. No ☐ 4 points

2. **What color is your urine most of the time?**

   A. Dark yellow ☐ 0 points
   B. Straw yellow ☐ 1 point
   C. Light yellow ☐ 2 points
   D. Clear ☐ 4 points

3. **How much water do you drink daily?**

   A. About one glass ☐ 0 points
   B. Two to three glasses ☐ 1 point
   C. Four to five glasses ☐ 3 points
   D. Six to eight glasses, or more ☐ 4 points

4. **How much caffeine do you consume daily?**

   A. I drink three or more caffeinated beverages throughout the day.
      ☐ 0 points
   B. I have two caffeinated beverages daily. ☐ 1 point
   C. I have about one caffeinated beverage daily. ☐ 4 points

5. **Do you pee a little when you cough, sneeze, laugh, or do routine physical activities, such as bending down, lifting, or walking?**

   A. Yes ☐ 0 points   B. No ☐ 4 points

6. **Do you have trouble controlling your urine flow or do you frequently wet your pants?**

   A. Yes ☐ 0 points   B. No ☐ 4 points

7. **How often do you feel "unsatisfied" after urinating, as though you still need to go but cannot?**

   A. Almost always ☐ 0 points
   B. More than half the time ☐ 1 point
   C. Less than half the time ☐ 2 points
   D. Never ☐ 4 points

8. **How often are you performing Kegel exercises?**

   A. Never ☐ 0 points
   B. A couple of times per week ☐ 1 point
   C. A few times per day ☐ 4 points

9. **Have you ever had kidney stones?**

   A. Yes ☐ 0 points   B. No ☐ 4 points

10. **How often do you strain to begin to urinate?**

    A. Almost always ☐ 0 points
    B. More than half the time ☐ 1 point
    C. Less than half the time ☐ 2 points
    D. Never ☐ 4 points

11. **How many times, on average, do you have to get out of bed at night to urinate?**

    A. Three or more times ☐ 0 points
    B. Twice ☐ 1 point
    C. Once ☐ 2 points
    D. Rarely or never ☐ 4 points

12. **In the last two weeks, how bothersome has trouble with urination been for you?**

    A. Very bothersome ☐ 0 points
    B. Sometimes bothersome ☐ 1 point
    C. A little bothersome ☐ 2 points
    D. Not bothersome at all ☐ 4 points

13. **Do you have trouble making it to the restroom in time when you have an urge to pee?**

    A. Yes ☐ 0 points   B. No ☐ 4 points

14. **Do you take cranberry supplements or drink cranberry juice regularly?**

    A. No ☐ 0 points   B. Yes ☐ 4 points

Scoring:

0–11: URGENT; see your doctor ASAP about the health of your urinary system.

12–22: DANGEROUS; change your hazardous urinary system tendencies immediately.

23–33: MODERATELY RISKY; start incorporating more of my suggestions for improved urinary tract health.

34–44: AVERAGE; you have room for additional change.

45–56: EXCELLENT; stay on this positive course.

There's no reason to be embarrassed if you have problems in the realm of your urinary system. It happens! There's also no need to be miserable with the symptoms. The organs within this system exist to help your body rid itself of toxins and waste. This is one of those systems that you can quickly and easily improve and protect. Take the steps, make the effort, and enjoy excellent urinary health well into ripe, old age.

CHAPTER 15

Cycle 3: 17 Day Plan

Y ou've now completed two cycles of this plan over 34 days, and you should be feeling great. In just a little over a month, if you've followed my simple suggestions, you've probably lost weight, built muscle, and improved your strength and endurance, not to mention all the improvements happening inside your body, right down to your cells. You've taken control of the five key factors of aging and effectively hit the pause button on Old Man Time. You are well on the path to living a long, healthy, happy life.

Cycle 3: Refine focuses on the intricacies of the third set of body systems we're working to improve, reinforce, and defend against the signs of aging. Those are the reproductive and urinary systems. Because some of the problems with these systems can be indicators of a larger problem in the body (such as how erectile dysfunction can be a sign of heart troubles), it is likely that as you've improved all the other body systems that we've covered, symptoms within these systems have already been alleviated. Still, there are more changes you can make that will fine-tune reproductive and urinary functions.

Before you begin Cycle 3, I want you to take a moment to give yourself a checkup. Look at my list on this page and mark all changes that apply to you.

CHECKUP: YOUR PROGRESS

I can work out longer and harder.

I breathe more deeply and calmly.

I am less forgetful.

My clothes are looser.

My bowel movements are regular.

I haven't caught a cold in the past month.

I notice more muscle definition.

I have a lot more energy.

I wake up feeling more rested.

Keep in mind as you go through Cycle 3 that if you scored low on any of the tests on these systems, you should continue doing the suggested strategies in those chapters even above and beyond what is mentioned in this 17 Day Plan.

Cycle 3: Refine Guidelines

1. Take the following supplements mentioned in the previous three chapters, but check your multivitamin and make sure you aren't doubling up on any of these:

   - Vitamin E—400 IU daily (do not exceed)
   - **Men Only:** Saw palmetto—as directed on bottle
   - Vitamin C—1,000 mg daily
   - Antioxidant vitamin (including beta-carotene)—as directed on bottle
   - Calcium—1,000 mg daily
   - Magnesium—400 mg daily
   - Cranberry—either two ounces of unsweetened cranberry juice daily or cranberry supplement as directed on bottle

2. Refine food guidelines:

   - If you are having urinary symptoms, avoid citrus fruits, caffeine, and sugary foods.
   - Include high-potassium foods daily, especially if you're prone to kidney stones.

3. Increase your NEAT every day on this plan. In fact, try to never remain continuously seated for an hour. Find ways to stand up and move around.

4. Take your cardio and strength training to a new level. Push yourself harder each day and get at least 30 minutes of heart-pumping exercise daily.

5. Perform 10 reps of Kegel exercises three times throughout each day in this cycle.

* *Ideas:* Do them while you're driving, waiting in line, sitting at the computer, or when you go to the bathroom.

6. You'll notice that I'm "prescribing" sex several times in this 17 Day Plan. This isn't permission to go crazy. This should be safe (both physically and emotionally) sex that you're having. If that simply isn't an option at the moment, masturbation is perfectly healthy and gives your body the same release that can lead to benefits for your reproductive system.

    * *Important:* Make sure you urinate before and immediately after sexual intercourse to help prevent bacteria from causing a urinary tract infection.

7. Look at your urine every day on this plan to make sure it's a normal, healthy color. (Refer to the urine color chart in chapter 14.) Remember that certain foods and medications will alter its color.

8. Don't neglect the anti-aging essentials just because you're now at Cycle 3. Staying hydrated is one of those key factors in overall health, and it certainly applies to both urinary and reproductive health and prevention of aging.

All of these guidelines apply to every day in this cycle even though you will be alternating days from the Restore and Rebuild plans. I'm simply showing you that it's possible to incorporate all the healthy suggestions from each of these systems into your day-to-day activities. There is nothing too challenging here—and the benefits all around are enormous.

So, are you ready to start Cycle 3: Refine? Let's go!

DAY 1

Follow **Rebuild Cycle** Day 1.

    Anytime: Call your doctor (women: call your gynecologist; men: call your urologist) if any of the following apply to you:

* *Women:* You have untreated menopause symptoms affecting your life.

* *Women:* You have general abdominal pain or pain with intercourse.

- *Women:* You are due for a mammogram or have noticed a change in your breasts.
- *Women/Men:* You have low libido (no sexual desire) or any other symptoms affecting your sex life.
- *Women/Men:* You have any urinary symptoms (going too often, waking up to pee often, pain during urination, weak stream, etc.).

DAY 2

Follow **Restore Cycle** Day 2.

DAY 3

Breakfast: Include one high-potassium food and one handful of blueberries.

- *Idea:* Combine ½ cup low-fat milk, one banana, one handful of blueberries, and one scoop of protein powder in the blender for a morning smoothie.

Lunch: Include at least one high-calcium food and one food from my anti-cancer cuisine list.

- *Idea:* Combine one serving of low-fat yogurt with ½ cup of strawberries.

Dinner: Include at least one food high in vitamin C.

- *Idea:* Try a veggie high in vitamin C, such as Brussels sprouts or bell peppers.

Anytime: Have sex with your partner, but remember to urinate before and immediately after.

DAY 4

Follow **Restore Cycle** Day 4.

DAY 5

Follow **Rebuild Cycle** Day 5.

DAY 6

Breakfast: Include one high-potassium food and one handful of blueberries.

- Drink one cup of coconut water and eat a bowl of oatmeal topped with blueberries.

Lunch: Include at least one food high in vitamin C in the form of a citrus fruit.

- *Idea:* Eat one grapefruit or tangerine along with your balanced lunch.

Dinner: Include at least one high-calcium food and one food from my anti-cancer cuisine list in chapter 12.

- *Idea:* Chop up fresh garlic cloves and sauté, then add one big handful of spinach and one big handful of kale. Heat just until wilted. Enjoy with one serving of light protein.

Anytime: Have sex with your partner, but remember to urinate before and immediately after.

DAY 7

Follow **Rebuild Cycle** Day 7.

DAY 8

Follow **Restore Cycle** Day 8.

DAY 9

Breakfast: Include at least one food high in vitamin C and one handful of blueberries.

- *Idea:* Combine several fruits and berries in a large bowl and have some of this for breakfast, then snack on this vitamin C powerhouse fruit salad over the next few days.

Lunch: Include one high-potassium food.

- *Idea:* Turn ½ of an avocado (yes! It's high in potassium) into a healthy guacamole with a squeeze of fresh lime juice, chopped cilantro, and some black pepper.

Dinner: Include at least one high-calcium food and one food from my anti-cancer cuisine list.

- *Idea:* Combine your three favorite beans with chicken broth and seasonings (including garlic) and make a three-bean soup. Grate low-fat cheddar cheese as your calcium topping.

DAY 10

Follow **Restore Cycle** Day 10.

DAY 11

Follow **Rebuild Cycle** Day 11.

DAY 12

Breakfast: Include at least one food high in vitamin C in the form of a citrus fruit.

Lunch: Include one high-potassium food and one handful of blueberries.

Dinner: Include at least one high-calcium food and one food from my anti-cancer cuisine list.

Anytime: Have sex with your partner, but remember to urinate before and immediately after.

DAY 13

Follow **Restore Cycle** Day 13.

DAY 14

Breakfast: Include at least one food high in vitamin C in the form of a citrus fruit.

Lunch: Include one high-potassium food and one handful of blueberries.

Dinner: Include at least one high-calcium food and one food from my anti-cancer cuisine list.

Anytime: Have sex with your partner, but remember to urinate before and immediately after.

DAY 15

Follow **Rebuild Cycle** Day 15.

DAY 16

Follow **Restore Cycle** Day 16.

DAY 17

Breakfast: Include at least one food high in vitamin C in the form of a citrus fruit.

Lunch: Include one high-potassium food and one handful of blueberries.

Dinner: Include at least one high-calcium food and one food from my anti-cancer cuisine list.

Anytime: Have sex with your partner, but remember to urinate before and immediately after.

How do feel? Energetic? Balanced? Focused, yet relaxed? Youthful? I hope you're so rejuvenated (not to mention proud of yourself) that you'll want to continue on with your new age-defying lifestyle for the rest of your life, which could be a very long time! I realize, as you should, that every day won't be perfect. And that's okay. When you wake up each morning, don't dwell on how you screwed up yesterday or how much you have to accomplish tomorrow. Focus on right now, today, because that's what's directly in front of you and those are the choices that matter at this very moment. Make the right ones, and you're investing in your ability to live 100 good—hopefully great—years.

Before we move on to our final cycle, retake the reproductive and urinary quizzes to measure your improvements.

PART FIVE

. . . .

Cycle 4: Renew

Following the advice and recommendations in the first three cycles of this book will help get you on the road to living well into old age while experiencing fewer of the rotten side effects often associated with aging. You'll likely look and feel better, too—who doesn't want that?

But there's more! The chapters in Cycle 4: Renew lay out strategies and an easy-to-follow 17 Day Plan related to other essential aspects of living a long, healthy, and happy life.

How does having more sex sound? How about getting a great night's sleep? Or reducing your exposure to potentially deadly toxins? I'll equip you with lifestyle secrets you'll love and want to access every day of your life.

You'll also discover that, in my estimation, there's a vital connection between longevity and how you choose to live your life on a daily basis. This is fundamental, folks. I'm talking about your overall lifestyle, and I think you'll be surprised by some of the information I reveal in this part of the book.

What are you waiting for? Let's keep moving toward 100 happy, healthy years.

CHAPTER 16

Clearing the Air on Toxins

There's quite a bit of hype out there about toxins these days. You may hear reports about how toxic buildups in the body can lead to cellulite, constipation, fatigue, and even autoimmune disease. Any number of horrible illnesses and health conditions have been attributed to toxins of late. Even more publicity is swirling around regarding the need to detoxify, cleanse, or purify your body. Some of this is pure propaganda created by people and companies just looking to profit off your fears, but I will concede the fact that your body and all its systems may be affected by the current levels of pollution, pesticides, contaminants, artificial substances in processed foods, and other types of toxins in today's world. Especially in high doses, toxins have the ability to speed up the aging process, disrupt hormones, suppress your immune system, and mangle your memory, and can sometimes even lead to cancer.

Here's the good news: Your body, especially when it's healthy, is extremely resilient. And if you're following the advice I've given you thus far, you're even improving on its ability to ward off toxic invaders. You can take this one step further by learning about the toxins in your environment and drastically reducing your overall exposure. I believe it's possible to reduce the impact of toxins on our health and pave the way to living 100 happy, healthy years.

Toxins 101

Some of the major toxins impacting our health include the following:

Indoor air pollution. Yes, you read that correctly. Pollution happens inside, too! And if you consider the fact that most Americans spend between 80 and 90 percent of their time indoors, this is a big deal. The Environmental Protection Agency believes indoor air pollution is one of the top five environmental threats to the American people. Studies conducted by the EPA also show that there are frequently two to five times higher levels of air pollution inside than there are outside. That's a lot! One big source of indoor pollution is industrial chemicals: compounds such as solvents, household products, fuels, glues, formaldehyde, and flame retardants, all found in many products used in industrial workplaces and in your home.

Outdoor air pollution. The term "outdoor air pollution" generally refers to a few environmental toxins including ozone, particles in the air, and nitrogen oxides. While hazy air is typically high in tiny particles of pollution, air that appears clean can also be loaded with particulate pollution that harms health. No doubt you're also aware that secondhand smoke can be harmful. Studies suggest it can damage not only your lungs but also your brain.

Indoor and outdoor pollution also includes exposure to heavy metals. No, I'm not talking about rock bands; I'm talking about real metals, such as aluminum, arsenic, cadmium, copper, iron, lead, mercury, and manganese, that get into our environment through various industrial and agricultural processes. In high amounts, all have been linked to neurological disorders. Most people absorb the metals through exposure to contaminated food, water, or air, or contact with the skin associated with the agriculture, manufacturing, or pharmaceutical industries or with products in the home.

AGEs. AGEs, or advanced glycation end-products, promote inflammation in your body, which you should know by now is no good! I think of AGEs as toxins because they truly are toxic to the overall health of all your body's systems. Your body can form these toxins in response to certain foods, based primarily on how the foods are prepared.

Pesticides. Pesticides refer to any substance used to kill or repel any type of biological pest: rodents, insects, spiders, mold, mildew, and the like. The invention of pesticides, in many ways, was a great thing. Pesticides enable farmers to keep their crops safe, which means greater production of food. They also keep various pests, including a wide variety of insects, mold, germs, mildew, weeds, and more, out of our daily lives.

Pesticides, however, are among the worst toxins. A study of people who worked in agriculture for 20 years or more found that those who had direct exposure to pesticides suffered up to five times greater likelihood of low scores on cognitive tests and double the likelihood of cognitive decline as those who did not come into close contact with pesticides.

How Toxins Can Age You

Exposure to environmental toxins has been pinpointed as one of the causes of aging, according to a recent article in *Clinics in Geriatric Medicine*. When regularly exposed to environmental toxins—which we all are—your body can get bogged down with chronic oxidative stress and free radicals may go on a rampage. Most organ systems can be harmed, but it's the brain that is perhaps most vulnerable. In fact, scientists believe that oxidative stress caused by toxins could be a major cause of Alzheimer's disease, other types of dementia, and Parkinson's disease.

Indoor air pollution can also contribute to and aggravate a slew of health problems, including asthma, eye irritation, memory problems, nausea, and even cancer. People with preexisting lung problems (such as chronic lung disease or asthma) are especially at risk. Symptoms include asthma attacks, coughing, inflammation in the airway, and other respiratory problems. We're all susceptible to indoor toxins, but people who have been overexposed to industrial chemicals are even worse off.

As for overexposure to heavy metals, these have been linked to neurological disorders. The chemicals are linked to acute symptoms such as blurred vision, slurred speech, and motor problems, and to increased risk for brain tumors and neurodegenerative diseases such as Parkinson's.

The Number-One Factor for Reducing Toxic Burden: Control Oxidative Stress

In previous chapters, I discussed oxidative stress, the damaging process that occurs when cell-damaging free radicals outnumber protective antioxidants, as one of the factors you can control. Prolonged oxidative stress causes free radicals to accrue, which can ultimately contribute to serious illnesses including cancer, diabetes, atherosclerosis, Alzheimer's disease, and rheumatoid arthritis. Oxidative stress intensifies with exposure to environmental toxins, so take measures daily to stamp this stress out.

If your score on the quiz in this chapter reveals above-normal exposure to toxins, I want you to add one more supplement to your antioxidant strategy: glutathione. Glutathione is a tripeptide, a protein made from three amino acids: cysteine, glutamic acid, and glycine. It protects cells against the damaging effects of oxidative stress and toxins and is particularly helpful in eliminating mercury, lead, cadmium, nickel, formaldehyde, pesticides, and other toxins from the body. Under oxidative stress, glutathione levels sharply decline, compromising your liver's ability to detoxify harmful substances. My recommendation: two to five grams daily.

Now, let me share some specific strategies for dealing with each of the major toxins that affect health and longevity.

The Hottest Detox Around

There are a lot of products, diets, juices, and clinics out there these days that claim to have the definitive answer on how to rid your body of all the toxins we encounter daily in order to reverse aging. But many of these trends can be dangerous. Here are some examples of potential dangers. Consider yourself warned!

Colonics: This is a type of "detox" that is essentially like getting a massive enema. During the procedure, the technician will pump up to 20 gallons of water into the colon to "clean" out the rectum. It really scares me to think about people having this done, especially patients who have any type of digestive disorder. So much can go wrong! The risks include perforation of your bowel wall, electrolyte imbalance and dehydration, infection from virus or bacteria, and the list goes on. Bottom line: In my medical opinion, colonics are not a smart idea.

Juice fasts: These may be all the rage, but I have my reservations. Simply put, if you're only consuming juice, with no solids at all, you're not getting the nutrients and enzymes your body needs. Therefore, you probably won't feel very good, and if you lose any weight, you're likely to gain it back relatively quickly. If you ask me, in general, whether I think juicing is a healthy way to consume fruits and vegetables, my answer is yes and no. If fresh juice is your *only* source of fruits and veggies, then you are missing out on most of the fiber because juicing removes the pulp, where much of the fiber comes from. But if fresh juice is part of your overall healthy diet and lifestyle, then I think it can be a terrific supplement. However, your body does not need you to do a juice fast for a week, or even a day.

Starvation diets: Do I really even need to comment on these? Any "detox" program that severely limits your caloric intake to let your organs "rest" is not going to be something I ever recommend. These can really mess around with your metabolism and other bodily functions. We were built to require fuel in the form of food. As for folks who think if they have a "bad eating day" filled with fast food, pizza, soda, or the like and then just starve themselves for a day or two afterward to make up for it . . . you know who you are . . . this is a terrible idea. If you screw up and detour a bit from your overall healthy lifestyle for a day or a weekend, just get back in the saddle the next day by returning to your normal, healthy diet. Starving yourself only makes matters worse, often forcing your body to store more fat.

So, you may ask, what do I think is the hottest, most revolutionary detoxification system in the world? Are you ready for this? It's the human body! That's right, folks, you were born fully equipped with a very powerful waste management system. When it's functioning properly, you are naturally able to rid yourself of most of the toxins you encounter as each system can adequately dump its waste into the urinary and digestive systems, which then release them out of your body. Your skin also acts as a way for your body to flush out waste—in the form of sweat! And to keep all of your systems functioning properly, I recommend you continue implementing the anti-aging essentials, all of which help your body filter and release toxins before they accumulate.

DRY SKIN BRUSHING

The evidence that dry skin brushing has any major health benefit is anecdotal, at best. You'll find some holistic practitioners who attribute all kinds of positive side effects to skin brushing, running the gamut from increased lymphatic drainage, a reduced appearance of cellulite, and general detoxification. Again, there's not a solid body of research indicating any of this. That said, it really can't hurt you, and at the very least it will help give your skin a healthy glow. Here's how to perform dry skin brushing:

Before taking a shower, when your skin is dry, use a dry skin brush or sponge (like ones you use in the shower, but keep this one dry at all times) to "brush" your skin. Try to get a brush with natural, not synthetic, bristles. It's best to start at your feet, moving the brush up toward your torso. Don't brush so hard that your skin turns red or irritated. Continue brushing, and work your way up your legs, torso, and arms. Do not perform dry skin brushing on any sensitive skin such as your face, nipples, and genitalia. When you're brushing the skin on your arms, go toward your armpits, not down toward your fingers. Just one quick sweep over the body is enough. As long as you're not irritating your skin, you can do this up to once a day.

Outdoor Air Pollution

Unless you've been living under a rock, you probably know that the quality of the air we all breathe in and out every day isn't what it once was. There are other types and sources of outdoor air pollution (including carbon monoxide and sulfur dioxide), but for our purposes, I'm going to focus on ozone, nitrogen oxide, and particulate matter.

You cannot see ozone pollution. Ozone, which is a gas comprised of three oxygen molecules, may not sound harmful on its surface. It's just oxygen, right? Well, when it gets into the tissues of your lungs, a reaction occurs that causes damage. This damage leads some people to experience trouble breathing, pain, inflammation, and more. It can land some high-risk folks in the hospital.

The presence of nitrogen oxides (N^2O) in the air has several causes, one of them being traffic-related pollution. Nitrogen oxides are a vital component in the formation of ozone, as well as smog. But it can cause health issues just on its own, including making us more vulnerable to various respiratory infections. Studies show that long-term exposure to traffic pollution might shorten our lives.

Particulate matter is another type of outdoor air pollution, and it is comprised of liquid and gas particles in our air. These can include sulfates, nitrates, metals, dust, and the like. There tend to be more particles in the air near industrial plants and major thoroughfares.

Together, these contributors to outdoor air pollution can be very dangerous to our respiratory systems, and also to other body systems. Some studies show that they can even increase our risk for heart attack (although not as much as other factors we've discussed), other heart-related health problems, and stroke. Furthermore, a large study has shown that over time, exposure to pollution, especially particulate matter, is linked to memory decline. Essentially, it's affecting our nervous system and brains, too—but you can fight it.

Supportive Strategies for Outdoor Air Pollution

Get informed. Your local news outlets typically report on the level of ozone in the air, especially during the summer, when levels tend to be higher. Air Quality Action Days, or Ozone Action days, occur when the levels of O^3 are quite high in the air, and you should take certain precautions (such as keeping windows closed, carpooling, and working out indoors) on these days, especially if you have a respiratory infection or condition. Children, people over the age of 65, diabetics, folks with heart conditions, and those who spend a lot of time outdoors are all at higher risk for suffering from the effects of ozone. On these days especially, I advise everyone—but especially my high-risk patients—to stay indoors during daylight hours as much as possible.

You can also take some steps to reduce your own toxin output. Consider carpooling, don't fill your gas tank until after the sun goes down (the gas vapor released won't have any sunlight to mix with and will release less pollution into the air), and don't mow your lawn (or wait until after dark, for the same reason). Even if you're a healthy individual, don't go outside for a run in the middle of the day on an Ozone Action Day. The faster you breathe, the more pollutants you're taking in. You know I'm a big fan of exercise, but your run can wait or you can work out indoors.

Supplement against air pollution. The fact is that air pollution is every-where. We discussed in the respiratory system chapter all the ways you can bolster the health of your lungs and airways, including practicing the anti-aging essentials, supplementing with B-complex vitamins to bal-ance methylation, and mastering deep breathing techniques. In addition, there is some evidence that omega-3 polyunsaturated fatty acids, espe-cially fish oils, can help by slowing the oxidative stress that occurs when we're exposed to air pollution. Also, we know the power of antioxidants, especially when it comes to eradicating free radicals, so boost your anti-oxidant intake when air pollution in your area is a problem.

Indoor Air Pollution

Poor indoor air quality is most commonly caused by gas or particulate matter being released by various sources indoors, and then it's worsened by poor ventilation, which means those gases and particles aren't diluted by enough outside air. So, what's in the air you're breathing inside? Obvi-ously, the answer depends on a lot of factors. First, is there a smoker liv-ing in your home? Secondhand smoke comes with all kinds of chemicals and poisons, many of which are carcinogens. Other sources are mold spores and pollens. Also, gases like radon, which is released naturally by the earth and can get into your home through foundation cracks, and carbon monoxide, which can be released by fuel-burning appliances, may be lurking in the air you breathe. Depending on when your home or office was built, formaldehyde and/or lead may be contributing to poor air quality and putting your health at risk. Pesticides are also sometimes a threat indoors.

If you're breathing in any of the above—which most of us are—you might be suffering from allergy symptoms (itchy eyes, nose, or throat, irritation, congestion, etc.). Other signs of problems are asthma-related issues like wheezing or shortness of breath. If you've been breathing pol-luted air on a regular basis for many years, the health effects could be det-rimental. If the pollutant isn't removed, people routinely exposed to it could suffer from serious heart and lung disease or cancer, and it could even prove fatal.

Supportive Strategies for Indoor Air Pollution

No smoking. This is one of the anti-aging essentials, but sometimes the smoke you're exposed to isn't because you're choosing to smoke. Remember to protect yourself when in public places, including hotels and rental cars. Always choose to sit away from smokers at a restaurant or bar, and request nonsmoking rooms and cars that haven't been smoked in previously.

Have your home tested. There are at-home tests you can purchase, or you can call upon a radon specialist in your area or possibly a home inspector (just make sure they are qualified). If the radon in your home is high, the EPA recommends that you have someone find and seal any cracks you may have, increase ventilation, and follow their other guidelines for reducing it. Once you have taken steps to reduce the radon content in your home, you should test again to make sure it has gone down and that it stays down. I recommend you also test for carbon monoxide and other pollutants. Speak with a home inspector about the tests that are typically done when someone is selling a home to make sure it's safe from mold, lead, asbestos, and other toxins. You don't need to be selling or buying a home to have these tests done; it's a smart move regardless to get this information and then work toward eliminating anything problematic.

Keep humidity at bay. If you live in a very humid area, consider using a dehumidifier (air conditioners naturally dehumidify the air as well), to reduce humidity inside. You want to keep general humidity low since water molecules in the air can increase the amount of pollutants, such as mold spores, that you're breathing. However, a dehumidifying device can do more harm than good if you allow it to get too dirty and it starts releasing these pollutants back into your air. Clean its filter regularly.

Air it out. If your home is tightly closed, with no air flow from the outside, you're not getting enough ventilation to reduce the overall amount of toxic particles inside. This can be resolved by simply keeping some windows open!

Find the source. While increasing ventilation will help dilute the presence of pollutants in your home, it's really better to locate the source. If you have leaky pipes, a crack in the foundation, or other structural issues, you should enlist the help of an expert to locate and reverse the flow of pollutants into your house.

Purify if possible. While air purifiers don't defend against noxious fumes or gases, many of them are effective at reducing the number of toxic particles in your home's air. There's a wide range of purifiers, so do your homework before purchasing one. Look for one that has a HEPA (high-efficiency particulate air) filter, because that will remove the tiniest of particles from the air. But just as with with a dehumidifier, you'll need to keep the filter clean so it doesn't get too full and start releasing the pollutants back into the air.

Bisphenol A (BPA)

Bisphenol A, or BPA, is a key chemical used in the manufacturing of plastic products, specifically polycarbonate plastics. It has been used in the plastic-making process since the 1960s. It's part of what makes these types of plastics strong and durable. Here are some of the many products that often contain BPA:

Food storage containers
Water bottles
Baby bottles
Cans for canned food
Plastic toys
Protective glasses
Medical tools
Dental sealants
Bicycle helmets
Various vehicle components
Adhesives
Various electronics
Compact discs

Some believe exposure to BPA can be linked to premature aging because of the cellular damage it inflicts, deadly diseases like breast cancer, or even behavioral problems in children who were exposed to it while in the womb. Others say more testing is needed before we can be sure BPA causes any harm to humans.

Rather than engage in an ongoing debate over this chemical compound, I'm instead going to give you my advice: Don't freak out, overreact, or become consumed with fear over this issue. Instead, follow my rules of thumb when it comes to BPA.

Supportive Strategies for BPA

Take inventory. First, I'd like you to become aware of BPA's presence in your household items, particularly the items with which you eat, drink, or store foods. Look in your cupboards, pantry, and refrigerator. Assess how many products you have from the above list. Do many of the foods you eat originate in a can? Are you microwaving food inside plastic containers on a regular basis, or putting plastic storage items in the dishwasher? Do you store all foods in plastic, or do you use a lot of glass containers? You don't need to go crazy here, but at least get a general idea.

Go fresh. It may mean taking trips to the grocery store or farmer's market more often, but there is enormous value in eating fresh food. Aim for eating 20 percent or less of your foods from a can because of the BPA content in the cans themselves. If you eat canned beans, consider buying them dry. Rather than tomato sauce from a can, consider buying a glass bottle.

Try glass. Purchase a few glass food storage containers, and throw out a few of your plastic ones. Try microwaving your food inside glass bowls, not plastic. I know there's a lot of convenience associated with plastic (it's lighter weight, less breakable, and cheaper), but the glass storage bowls you can find at the grocery store these days are great and very durable. And they last for ages, so you won't have to buy them again and again.

Hand wash your plastics. Since there's a possibility that the extreme heat inside your dishwasher (and microwave) can break down the various chemical compounds in the plastic, I advise hand washing all plastic food storage containers.

Look for BPA-free. Several companies have answered the call of concern by creating BPA-free water bottles, baby bottles, and more. I'm not saying to throw all your plastics out and replace them with BPA-free ones. But, for example, if you drink water from the same plastic bottle every day, consider replacing that with a BPA-free one.

Advanced Glycation End-Products (AGEs)

Remember our earlier discussion of glycation? It's one of the five controllable factors of aging. AGEs are chemicals in the body that occur when glucose molecules bond together with fat, proteins, or even DNA. This is not good, because it causes a sort of tangled-up mess of molecules, which have an adverse effect on your various organs, including your heart. AGEs are more likely to occur when foods, especially fatty foods, have been cooked at an extremely high temperature, such as when they are fried. So, all those French fries and that fried chicken can be big culprits in the formation of AGEs in your body. The same is true for foods that are broiled or grilled at high temps for long periods of time.

One study showed that a diet low in AGEs reduced inflammation, and thus the risk for developing heart disease. Here's how you can achieve that.

Supportive Strategies for AGEs

Vary your food preparations. When it comes to reducing your risk for eating foods that will increase inflammation, glycation, and other dangerous processes, there are some easy tricks to remember. Studies have shown that foods, especially animal fats and proteins, release fewer AGEs if they are cooked using moist heat instead of dry heat. Try boiling, steaming, poaching, or stewing the majority of your foods. I'm not saying to throw out your grill! I'm just saying not to prepare every meal on it. In the case of fruits and vegetables, eating them raw is always a great idea because they generally offer the most nutrients when uncooked.

Ditch the drive-thru. Studies show that some of the worst offenders when it comes to creating AGEs in your body are items you're likely to see on a menu (one dollar or otherwise) at any number of fast-food chains, pizza parlors, and hot-dog stands, because these are the ones that tend to be deep fried or charbroiled. Yes, I know, many fast-food chains are making an effort to carry healthier food choices. But if you really wanted some apple slices or low-fat milk, couldn't you just as easily hop into a grocery store and pick up these items? You'd spend less money, too. Most people I know who frequent the drive-thru window rattle off excuses like "I just don't have time to prepare a meal," or "It's just so convenient," or "I really don't go that often." But do you really want to sacrifice your health and longevity just because you can't resist having the cheeseburger and French fry combo every day? Is it really worth it?

The risk doesn't begin and end at the drive-thru window, however. If you eat out at any type of restaurant on a regular basis, I urge you to be cognizant of your choices. Just because you're at a fine dining establishment doesn't mean every item on the menu is fine for your health. Consider asking for a crudités platter of chopped veggies instead of a basket of buttery bread, ordering wraps instead of carb-heavy sandwiches, selecting steamed veggies over fried, asking the waiter to point out the healthiest items on the menu, or checking out the menu online before you go and deciding exactly what you'll order. You don't have to change your routine in order to make healthier food choices.

Pesticides

As you can imagine, since pesticides are designed to kill pests, they can also harm us if improperly used or abused. Some pesticides get into the produce we're consuming, and ultimately into our bodies. According to the Environmental Working Group, pesticides have been associated with damage to the nervous system, certain types of cancer, and endocrine problems.

Studies have linked the presence of pesticides in children's blood to attention or cognition issues. Specifically, one study based on research collected by the National Health and Nutrition Examination Survey discovered that even children who ingest what are considered to be "typical" amounts of pesticides from food show a higher risk of developing attention-deficit/hyperactivity disorder (ADHD).

You don't want to interact with pesticides more than necessary because they can cause a range of harmful effects including skin and eye irritation and damage to the nervous system, and in larger doses they can even be deadly, so here are some simple solutions to "detox" your body and your life as much as possible from the potentially harmful effects of pesticides.

Supportive Strategies for Pesticides

Clean out the cleaning supplies. The American Association of Poison Control Centers reports that household cleaners are one of the most common causes of poisonings in America. Yet it is such a simple factor to eradicate! This may make me sound like a hippie, but why not try less toxic disinfectants such as baking soda, lemon juice, white vinegar, hydrogen peroxide, or even rubbing alcohol? The first step is to make sure all of your cleaning supplies are put away in a cool, dry place that is not accessible to children or pets. Secondly, I want you to wear rubber gloves any time you are handling these products. Also, pull out all the cleaning supplies you have and see which ones you can replace with less toxic cleaners like those I listed above. Because people are becoming increasingly aware of this problem, there are many new cleaning products on the market that are less toxic. Breathing fewer toxic fumes and getting less of those materials on your skin is always a good thing.

Eat organic. Yes, I know organic fruits and vegetables are more expensive. But it might be worth the money to buy at least some foods from the organic section in the grocery store. Experts have evaluated many types of produce and found that there are specific ones you should aim to purchase organic because the commercial versions of these tend to test higher in pesticides, most likely because they have thinner peels or skins, allowing pesticides to enter more easily. Remember, this applies to frozen produce too! Here's the list of fruits and veggies you should aim to purchase organic:

Apples
Celery
Strawberries
Blueberries
Peaches
Nectarines

Grapes
Sweet bell peppers
Potatoes
Spinach
Lettuce
Kale/Collard greens

Consider shopping at local farmers' markets. That's where you're likely to get the freshest produce, straight off the farm. But still ask whether the food is grown organically.

The following fruits and vegetables typically test lower in pesticides, most likely because they are protected by a thicker, more impervious skin. These are probably okay to purchase non-organic:

Onions
Sweet corn
Pineapples
Avocado
Asparagus
Sweet peas
Mangoes
Eggplant
Cantaloupe
Kiwi
Cabbage
Sweet potatoes
Mushrooms

Try natural pesticides. If you have your own garden, especially if you plant fruits and veggies, I encourage you to try some natural ways to kill bugs and weeds. Try spraying white vinegar on your weeds. And if you know what type of pest you're trying to kill, do a little research into what natural products are most likely to kill them. In general, it's worth grinding up some garlic and sprinkling it around you garden, as well as cayenne pepper, cinnamon, and cloves. There are several organic, nontoxic bug and pest killers on the market, too. Plus, all-natural anti-pest solutions will keep pets safer.

What's Your Body's Toxic Burden?

Answer each question honestly; give yourself the designated points for each answer. Add up your total and score yourself.

1. **Do you ever microwave your food in plastic containers?**

    A. Yes ☐ 0   B. No ☐ 4

2. **Do you drive in heavy traffic most days of the week?**

    A. Yes ☐ 0   B. No ☐ 4

3. **Do you eat fast-food or at restaurants several times a week?**

    A. Yes ☐ 0   B. No ☐ 4

4. **Do you primarily consume organic fruits and veggies?**

    A. No ☐ 0   B. Yes ☐ 4

5. **Do you use commercial household cleaners without gloves on a regular basis?**

    A. Yes ☐ 0   B. No ☐ 4

6. **Do you currently smoke or are you regularly exposed to secondhand smoke?**

    A. Yes ☐ 0   B. No ☐ 4

7. **Do you regularly use non-organic bug spray or weed killer in your home and garden, or do you have a regular pest control service?**

    A. Yes ☐ 0   B. No ☐ 4

8. **Does your occupation expose you to industrial chemicals (paint, solvents, industrial cleaners, harsh chemicals, etc.)?**

    A. Yes ☐ 0   B. No ☐ 4

9. **Do you live in or near a highly polluted area?**

    A. Yes ☐ 0   B. No ☐ 4

10. **Is your home well ventilated, or do you use an air purifier?**

    A. No ☐ 0   B. Yes ☐ 4

11. **Have you ever had your home tested for radon or carbon monoxide?**

    A. No ☐ 0   B. Yes ☐ 4

12. **Do you store foods mostly in glass or other non-plastic containers?**

    A. No ☐ 0   B. Yes ☐ 4

13. **Do you eat more canned food than fresh food?**

    A. Yes ☐ 0   B. No ☐ 4

14. **Do you prepare the vast majority of your foods at high heat, such as grilling, broiling, or frying for long periods of time?**

    A. Yes ☐ 0   B. No ☐ 4

Scoring:

0–11: URGENT; take steps today to change your habits pertaining to toxicity.

12–22: DANGEROUS; change any behavior that could increase your toxic burden.

23–33: MODERATELY RISKY; do more of my suggestions for lowering your overall exposure to toxins.

34–44: AVERAGE; you have room for additional change.

45–56: EXCELLENT; stay on this positive course.

If you didn't score too well on this quiz, don't panic. You are not doomed to experience all the worst possible repercussions of your encounters with toxins. It just means you need to step up your attempts to eradicate as many toxic and harmful materials from your life as possible. If you are elderly, have someone who is elderly in your home, or are raising kids, I recommend you make some immediate changes. As we get older, our bodies become more vulnerable to various types of toxins. The same applies to children; their delicate systems can't as easily rid themselves of harmful substances.

Reducing your exposure to potentially toxic materials is an important factor in your journey toward 100 happy, healthy years. You can do it!

CHAPTER 17

HOW You Live → How LONG You Live

Despite what you may be thinking by now, the secret to living a long, vibrant life isn't *just* about eating vegetables, taking supplements, moving your body, and not smoking. My oldest and happiest patients know that life is about balance. It's about choosing, each and every day, to live life to the fullest. See and experience the world around you, try new things, make new connections, have fun. Those may not sound like the typical prescriptions from your M.D., but they're just as fundamental to living 100 happy, healthy years as drinking water and breathing air.

The way you look at the world impacts every aspect of how you live your life. Do you look at life as something to be survived, or do you believe in thriving from day to day? Do you have passions and seek them out, or do you sit on the sidelines and watch while others pursue their dreams? Your state of mind doesn't just determine if you're in a good mood on any given day; it impacts the health of your entire body. Sometimes it's hard to see the glass as half-full, but the benefits of viewing life that way are endless. So stop any negative, pessimistic thoughts in your head (easier said than done sometimes, I know) and just accept that a long, healthy, happy life is right in front of you if you work at it. So reach out and grab it!

More Sex for a Longer Life

Here are some doctor's orders you should be happy to receive: Have sex several times a week. Many people view a roll in the hay as a "want," but it's actually a "need," because sex is one of the keys to living 100 happy, healthy years. Some recent medical statistics show that (safe) sex at least three times a week can add nearly two years to your life because it increases your heart rate and the flow of blood throughout your body. Three times a week isn't enough for you? Then do it every day and your life expectancy increases by eight years! Get hitched and things get even better: Sex, within the context of marital intimacy, can add another four years to your life.

These studies confirm what I see in my own practice. Let me introduce you to Dottie and Frank, who have been married for over 60 years (imagine!). They are now in their 80s, with a sex life that would rival most 18-year-olds'.

What's their secret? Well, they're always experimenting, keeping their sexual relationship fresh and exciting. They have sex three times a week, but just as important, they keep up the romance. Unlike many of my male patients in this elderly age group, Frank doesn't need Viagra or any other erectile dysfunction drugs. All this couple needs is the power of their passion for each other. I expect them to live 100 happy, healthy years—they're already close, so it's clear they're doing something right.

Sex can help you feel youthful and healthy when practiced safely and within the confines of a committed relationship. (I'm not here to give a lecture about sexually transmitted diseases. Suffice it to say that promiscuous sex with multiple partners can be very dangerous.)

Here's a look at the multiple benefits:

Sex helps you live longer. One of the reasons that sex feels so good is because of the chemicals released during intercourse. These include dehydroepiandrosterone (DHEA), a building block of testosterone, a sex hormone, which helps to repair and heal tissue. Another is human growth hormone, which helps your body stay youthful.

Sex boosts your immunity. Studies conducted at Wilkes University in Pennsylvania indicated that having intercourse one or two times a week raises the level of an antibody called immunoglobin A (IgA) by as much as one-third. IgA helps fortify your immune system because it binds itself to germs that enter the body.

Sex helps prevent prostate cancer. Yes, gentlemen, you read that correctly. Studies show that men who have frequent ejaculations in their 20s can have a significantly lower risk of prostate cancer as they age. Your 20s have come and gone? It's not too late for sex to help you. Another survey by the National Cancer Institute demonstrated that middle-aged men who average 21 ejaculations a month have a 33 percent lower risk for prostate cancer, compared to those with only four to seven ejaculations.

Sex is a painkiller. Pain of any variety puts a damper on living 100 quality years. But here comes sex to the rescue! Sex works as an analgesic in your body (much like aspirin or acetaminophen). During orgasm, the brain opens the floodgates of the hormone oxytocin, which acts as a natural painkiller. So before you head to the medicine cabinet, consider engaging in sex with your partner to treat pain from arthritis, migraines, or just simple achiness.

Sex makes you happy. Remember what I said about sexual intercourse releasing the hormone DHEA? Well, that hormone acts as a mood enhancer or natural antidepressant. In other words, sexually released DHEA is an "upper," especially for women.

Sex protects heart health. In research that was aimed at identifying sex as a risk factor for heart attack in older patients, just the opposite proved true! This English study followed men for 20 years and found that not only was there no increased risk for strokes in elderly couples who engage in sex, but that if they had sex at least twice a week, they'd cut their risk of having a fatal heart attack in half.

Why was this? Easy. Sex increases circulation, reduces blood pressure, and has overwhelming benefits for the heart. So next time you want to do something good for your heart (emotionally and physically), jump into the sack with your partner!

My 100 Healthy Years Prescription

The everyday hustle and bustle of our busy lives can reduce time for intimacy. Do not let your schedule become so overrun that there is not enough time for quality sex. It is easy to let the world get the best of you and your partner get the rest of you, but schedule time to have sex when you are not exhausted. And get creative! Leave flirty notes for your partner, or create a secret code for your calendars. You may not think of sexual intimacy as an element of your overall physical health, but trust me, it is.

Companionship Is Key

What's the point of living 100 years if you're all by yourself? Depriving yourself of human interaction is just as bad an idea as not drinking enough water. Believe it or not, people who characterize themselves as socially connected tend to have lower blood pressure and stronger immunity. Plus, the more you plug in to your community of friends and family, the higher your cognitive performance. Not convinced? A study on over 300,000 people at Brigham Young University and the University of North Carolina showed that spending time with friends not only has health benefits, but it decreases your risk of an early death.

So, what does being plugged in mean to you? Here are just a few examples of ways you can increase your social interaction, and all the great health benefits you'll get in exchange.

Love is a powerful drug. Patients who have survived a serious disease, such as cancer, will tell you that they couldn't have gotten through it without the love and support of their families. There's scientific evidence to back that notion. A study conducted at the University of Iowa on patients with ovarian cancer showed that the participants who reported having the most solid relationships also had something else going for them. They may have had the best chance of beating their cancer, thanks to increased activity of white blood cells in the areas surrounding their tumors. Long "love" story short: Being in love and having dear friends boosts your health.

Now what if you don't have family close by? For one thing, close friends count. Friendship and involvement in social activities may protect you from depression and give you a healthier life. There's nothing like a close friend or confidant with a shoulder to cry on to help you deal with life's stresses, including an illness. We simply thrive better with a close circle of friends who care.

Nurture your friendships and enlarge your circle of friends, if necessary. Join a house of worship, a book club, a singles group, or a volunteer group, to name just a few ways to meet people. I don't need a research study to tell you what you already know: Friendship may be the best medicine of all.

Pay it forward. Helping others can help you reap health rewards. People who volunteer their time to help others generally enjoy a lowered risk of heart disease, reduced rates of depression, and increased longevity. Talk about a win-win! Others benefit directly from your kindness, and your health and sense of well-being improve.

You may have considered volunteering but don't know where to begin. Here's how:

Analyze your talents. What are you good at? If you are handy with tools, perhaps you can help fix things around the homes of elderly or disabled persons. If you have medical skills, perhaps you might volunteer at a low-income clinic or hospital. If you have human resources talents, maybe you can help out-of-work people create their résumés. Your talents can be enormously helpful to many organizations.

Consider your passions. What do you love doing? Volunteer in an area that gives you joy. Say you love to read; perhaps you could read to people who are visually impaired. Let's suppose you love working with children; you could volunteer to teach a Sunday school class. Maybe you love sports. Why not volunteer to coach a team for underprivileged kids? The more passionate you are about your volunteer activity, the more you bring to it when you step up to the plate.

Whatever you choose to do, remember it's not about you. Yes, you'll reap psychological and physical health benefits, but you've got to keep in mind that you are doing this for others, not only for yourself.

Embrace your inner extrovert. I love hanging out with friends and family, but not everyone enjoys going out, entertaining, and mixing and mingling as much as I do. But even if it's hard for you to muster up the energy to socialize, it's worth it, I promise! If you need some hard evidence, Australian researchers conducted a study with elderly people, and the social butterflies of the group were less likely to die over a 10-year period when compared to the people with the fewest friends.

Extroverted folks also enjoy a lower risk of a dementia diagnosis. Researchers in Sweden at the Karolinska Institutet studied a group of more than 500 elderly people (78+ years old), and discovered that the most gregarious of the participants had a 50 percent lower chance of losing brain function later in life. An added bonus: This same group reported that they tended to not experience stress. Moral of the story: Party down to stress less and live long!

INSPIRATION FROM SOMEONE WHO KNOWS

Dovie is one of my patients who just so happens to be 93 years old. She recently shared her secret for aging so gracefully with me. Throughout all her life, she's been surrounded by people. She joked that even after she retired from the U.S. Postal Service and then from her second career at a steel plant, she never really stopped working because her relatives, who adore her, kept her busy. They loved to come over and visit, so she was always cooking or caring for someone. Dovie also made plenty of time for volunteering at her church, where she worked with the elderly congregants who were less fortunate than she. She thinks it's this ongoing positive human interaction that has kept her going all these years. She woke up every single day with a sense of purpose and knowing that she would be engaging with others who either counted on her or loved her—or both!

That's the formula that has worked for Dovie for 10 decades. What is your formula?

My 100 Happy, Healthy Years Prescription

No matter your current age, companionship and social interaction are very important ingredients in the recipe for a long, fulfilling life. You don't have to be the most popular neighbor on the block or host extravagant parties to experience the benefits of engaging in your community. It can be as simple as volunteering at your local homeless shelter one night a week or playing cards with a friend on the weekends. We're social creatures, right? Don't get so caught up in the daily grind that you forget to have some fun with loved ones!

Sleep Your Way to 100 Happy, Healthy Years

Sleep is something I know a lot about, not only from the medical standpoint but from my own experiences. As a doctor, I have a long history of missing sleep. As an intern and resident at a busy hospital, I was required to work all day, all night, and through the following day before I could get to bed. Sometimes I did this every second or third night—brutal!

Obviously that wasn't the ideal state in which to be making life-or-death decisions for others, nor did it do my overall health any favors.

A chronic lack of sleep could cut your life short. You've probably heard that we should all be getting eight hours of sleep every night, but lots of new research suggests adults live longer if they get six to eight, which is more realistic for many of us.

Getting adequate sleep is always important, but even more so as we age. Just as you needed extra zzz's as a teenager, when you reach your latter years, your body once again craves extra sleep to recharge. Rather than obsess over the sum of hours you've slept, focus on your "sleep quality"— how well you sleep. For example, instead of going to bed and sleeping only six out of eight hours while spending the rest tossing and turning, it's more "efficient" to go to bed for six hours and actually sleep for those six hours. If you're not an A-plus sleeper, here's my prescription to improve the quality of your snooze.

My 100 Happy, Healthy Years Prescription

Sleep with soft ear plugs. They'll muffle ambient noise while allowing you to still hear loud, high sounds such as alarms and doorbells.

Try sleeping with eyeshades. They can block even the brightest light source. Some come with lavender flower filling that provides soothing aromatherapy.

Listen to white noise. Special sleep machines emit soothing sounds from nature or white noise to mask other sounds.

Distract your busy brain. Many of my patients tell me the moment their head hits the pillow, a million thoughts begin swirling around and sleep feels like a million miles away. So, before you hit the sack, try reading (the more boring the book, the better), watching TV, or listening to soothing music. Do this pre-sleep routine outside of the bedroom, and then drag yourself to bed when you can hardly keep your eyes open anymore. Your brain should be switched into "off" mode by the time you're between the sheets.

No booze within three hours of bedtime. Although alcohol can some-times make you feel sleepy, it ultimately stands in the way of a healthy balance between REM and non-REM sleep. In other words, even if you feel like you're sleeping deeply, the alcohol is actually messing with your sleep rhythms. Furthermore, we know alcohol has a negative effect on a myriad of medications, so you may experience drug interactions that keep you awake.

No caffeine after 3 p.m. Avoid coffee and other caffeinated beverages, since caffeine is a stimulant that may keep you awake.

Use caution with sleep drugs. Be careful with both prescription and over-the-counter sleep medications because you can easily get dependent on them. Plus, sleeping pills can cause daytime drowsiness and impair mem-ory, and they're also associated with falls. Over-the-counter medications often contain diphenhydramine (Benadryl), which can cause confusion in some elderly people.

Beware of side effects. If you're on a medication that is causing insomnia, speak to your doctor about finding an alternative to that med. The fol-lowing common drugs are apt to cause insomnia: steroids, beta blockers, decongestants, diet pills, thyroid medications, and asthma meds.

Keep a sleep routine. Go to bed at about the same time each night, and get up at the same time in the mornings, even on the weekends. Of course there will be an exception here and there when you're out too late and indulge by hitting "snooze," but day in and day out, do your best to keep your sleep hours consistent.

Other sleep tips for longer life: If you have trouble going to sleep at night, create a pre-sleep ritual like a warm bath, a light (protein) snack, or maybe some meditation. And create a cozy sleeping environment: total darkness and silence, a comfortable (not too warm or cold) tempera-ture, and an uncluttered bedroom. If you can't fall asleep within 15 min-utes of crawling under the covers, get out of bed and do something relaxing. Then, try again. If you're a napper, schedule naps for early in the day so they don't disrupt your overnight sleep patterns.

SLEEP ALERT: CALL YOUR DOCTOR

Does your partner go to bed wearing noise-reducing earphones to muffle the sound of your nightly chainsaw-like snoring routine? Even if you don't want to admit it, if you're regularly snoring or gasping during sleep, or you wake up every morning feeling over-the-top exhausted despite apparently sleeping soundly, you may have sleep apnea, a common sleep disorder. With sleep apnea, the airway collapses during sleep and keeps air from reaching the lungs. The sufferer will snore loudly, but with pauses in breathing. If you have sleep apnea, you'll feel perpetually exhausted. And you might have headaches, moodiness, and poor concentration. A dangerous side effect is that because sufferers don't sleep well at night, they may fall asleep at the wrong time—like at a stoplight. Untreated, sleep apnea can cause high blood pressure, a forerunner of heart attacks and strokes. The most common treatment is a breathing machine and mask called a CPAP. It generates air pressure, which flows through a tube into the mask. This keeps the airway open during sleep. Folks with the highest risk of sleep apnea tend to be overweight or obese, but you can still have it if your weight is normal.

If the symptoms above are disturbing your slumber (and your life), see your doctor. There are sleep disorder clinics that can properly diagnose you, and there are several different treatment options to consider.

Take Fewer Pills

I know this sounds a little depressing, but the truth about aging is that we often have more medical problems and we take more meds as a result. My sincere hope is that you won't fall in the crowded category of elderly people who swallow handfuls of pills every day just to get by. That's because with those extra pills come extra (and unwelcome) health issues.

And then there are patients like Edward, who is in his 90s and takes no prescription drugs! I can barely call him a patient, because he is in such great health that I rarely see him. But I remain his family doctor.

Edward admits, and I agree, that genetics have played a part in his long life. But he has put in effort as well. He enjoys a glass of wine daily (he prefers cabernets and has brought me several bottles of his favorites over the years. Thanks, Edward!). The only pills he takes daily are a multivitamin, baby aspirin, and glucosamine, a natural supplement, for his arthritis. He gets annual checkups with me. He drinks eight to 10 glasses of water daily and keeps up his regular hobby of painting. I'd say this guy does just about everything it takes to enjoy 100 happy, healthy years—including the fact that he takes no prescription drugs.

Yes, Edward is in the minority. These days, many older folks (and sometimes not-so-old folks) sit around with friends and discuss all the various pills they take and their health problems. Sounds like really riveting conversation, huh? With most elderly people, it's dangerous to ask a question like "How are you?" because they might just go on and on about all their health problems. Not so with Edward, who'd rather talk about his passions and share his enthusiasm with you.

I'll be the first to say that medicines do save lives, but very few are completely free of risks or side effects, which is why I push prevention over pills. The more drugs you take together, the greater the risk for side effects and harmful interactions.

People these days seem to be taking so many drugs that experts have even labeled the phenomenon: polypharmacy. It essentially means "multiple drugs." It applies to more and more people as they seek out several doctors for various ailments and end up with many different prescriptions, all of which could have contraindications, especially when the doctors are not working closely together. I see polypharmacy more commonly in older people, who tend to have more chronic conditions that call for drug treatments. It's not necessarily the patients' fault—they're just doing what they're told. But I'm here to tell you that you've got to take control over what you're putting in your body, no matter who told you to do it. You need to ask questions and get informed.

Polypharmacy isn't the only problem. Aging also changes the body's ability to tolerate and process medications: Muscle tissue and fluid levels drop, fat tissue increases, liver mass shrinks, and kidney function declines. The net effect can be a huge decline in quality of life.

Get this: We recently received prescription drug use reports from the Federal Centers for Disease Control and Prevention. They estimated that nearly half of all Americans take at least one prescription drug and one in six Americans takes at least three. That's a lot of visits to the local pharmacy.

But what does it mean for your health? For instance, let's say you're taking six different drugs. Perhaps you're taking a statin for cholesterol, an antidepressant, blood pressure medication, an anti-inflammatory, an occasional anti-anxiety prescription, and an allergy medication. Take all six of those drugs, and you've got yourself 80 percent odds of *at least* one drug interaction, which we call a contraindication. Let's take it up to eight drugs (maybe add in some baby aspirin and an antibiotic), and now your chance is 100 percent.

Many people are concerned about the side effects of their prescription drugs. Just listen to those prescription drug ads as they carefully list side effect after side effect at record speed at the end of a commercial, and you'll probably get a little nervous! Doctors are also concerned, which is why we tell you to come back for routine appointments and blood tests. We want to keep an eye on how you're doing with each medication. There can be subtle (or not-so-subtle) changes that alert us to the need for adjusting dosage or changing the drug altogether. If you think you are having a side effect from a medication, discuss it with your doctor. But don't ever just stop taking the pill at your discretion or refuse to take it in the first place. This is a decision you need to make together with your physician.

Meet with your family doctor about all the pills (including supplements) you're taking. Get on the same page so you can work together to create or modify a plan that works for you. You may be surprised by how many alternatives there are for most prescriptions. Even if you think you're doing well on a particular medication, many treatments should change as time passes. I get it that you may not want to rock the boat if your health seems to be in check, but sometimes less can be better. I have helped cut the number of drugs a patient is taking by as much as 50 percent by adding lifestyle strategies such as increased cardiovascular exercise or a specific diet. There is no magic number of pills that constitutes polypharmacy, but if you feel you are taking too many drugs, you should probably have your drug regimen checked out by your doctor. Perhaps pills can help you feel better in the "now," but in the long run, it's better to rely less on pills and more on prevention.

My 100 Happy, Healthy Years Prescription

If you're routinely taking prescription meds, I have this advice for you: Make an appointment with your physician to discuss the following.

1. Any questions you have about the drugs' purpose, side effects, and contraindications.

2. Everything you're taking. And I mean everything—herbs, vitamins, supplements, recreational drugs, alcohol, and prescriptions. (Doctors aren't judging you—they just need all the information in order to guide you on what to do.) The reason for this is because certain supplements and herbs can actually have dangerous effects when taken with prescriptions. I ask my patients to put all prescription and over-the-counter drugs they are using, have used in the last month, or are likely to use in a bag and bring them along. That way, I can evaluate the drugs, strengths, and dosages.

3. Whether your "pill load" is too high. In other words, are you having trouble taking as many pills as you've been prescribed? Maybe you can't remember to take them all or they're too difficult to swallow. If so, your doctor may be able to reduce your total number of prescriptions.

4. Cost. If you have trouble affording everything you've been prescribed, it's worth bringing up. Obviously your doctor isn't your accountant, but he or she may be aware of cheaper alternatives or programs that can help.

5. Any new aches, pains, sweats, or any other symptoms you're having since starting a new drug.

If you want your body to perform at its peak and start living 100 *great* years, work with your doctor on your medication routine and needs. But just take the medications you *really* need.

Eat Less

Weight is an ever-expanding topic. I'm talking about body fat, particularly of the visceral variety. This is the deadly fat that surrounds your organs, not the kind just under the skin. Know this: If you carry too much fat on your body, especially around your middle, you may be shortening your life. For health and longevity, it pays to be thin.

But let me be clear about the heading of this section. When I say "eat less," I'm talking about your portions. As you surely know by now, I'm a huge believer in fueling your body with the healthiest, most natural foods available. I want you to eat foods that are the richest in nutrients.

Do I believe in counting calories? I believe you should at least be aware of them.

The research shows that eating 1,400 to 2,000 (healthy) calories per day seems to improve the functioning of your heart. Indeed, if you do this, your heart could perform at a level similar to that of when you were 15 years younger than you are today. A low-calorie diet, even in folks who aren't obese, can also lead to changes in metabolism and body chemistry that have been linked to better health and longer life, researchers have reported.

Let's talk for a moment about the Japanese people, specifically the ones who reside in Okinawa. They're known to live long, healthy lives, especially compared to people from other countries like the United States. Now, I'm not discounting the potential genetic advantages they may have, such as some built-in natural resistance to inflammation (which we know can lead to a whole host of serious illnesses). But did you know that some Japanese people follow a tradition called "Hara Hachi Bu," which means "Eat until you are 80 percent full"?

I love this concept and I wish all of my patients would practice it. Here's why: After your last bite of a meal, it takes a full 20 minutes before you're going to feel full. That's because it takes that long for your stomach to tell your brain that it's time to stop eating because you're at maximum capacity! If you kept eating past that point, as so many people do, later you'd feel overly full, bloated, and downright gross. Have you ever heard the term "food coma"? This is how you avoid it!

MORE FIBER? SWEET!

Most Americans eat 14 to 17 grams of fiber per day. But by adding another 10 grams a day, you could reduce your risk of dying from heart disease by 17 percent, according to a Netherlands study. Dietary fiber helps reduce total and LDL ("bad") cholesterol, improve insulin sensitivity, and boost weight loss.

Here's my sweet and simple fix: Top your oatmeal (½ cup dry oatmeal has 4 grams of fiber) with one cup of raspberries (8 grams of fiber), and you get 12 grams of fiber in just one meal. Other fiber-rich foods are ½ cup of 100-percent bran cereal (8.8 g), ½ cup of cooked lentils (7.8 g), ½ cup of cooked black beans (7.5 g), one medium sweet potato (4.8 g), and one small pear (4.3 g).

My 100 Happy, Healthy Years Prescription

Regardless of what diet you follow, try to eat 25 percent fewer calories than normal. First, keep a three-day food record. Write down everything you eat and your estimated calorie count for each of the three days. Then look for ways to slash the calories by 25 percent. Don't forget to reduce sugar, unhealthy fats, and processed foods, and opt for high-fiber choices, particularly veggies and lean proteins. And listen to your body—when you're just about 80 percent full, but not completely satisfied, push the plate away. Follow these guidelines and you will lose weight. Your blood pressure will fall. Your heart will be healthier. You will live longer. It really is as simple as it sounds, folks!

Does Your Attitude Need Adjusting?

Even if you won the genetic lottery and you've got the type of body that seems to never get sick, bounces back instantly after injury, and looks 25 years old even though you're 50, you could still cut your life short just by having the wrong attitude. Now, I'm no psychologist and I don't pretend to be one, but I know what I see in my own patients, in my own life, and in the medical journals. The folks with the most positive outlook on life are the ones who tend to be the healthiest and live the longest, and they're the ones who tend to beat the odds when they do get sick.

Margaret is the perfect example of this. She's a patient of mine who received the bad news of a breast cancer diagnosis well into her 80s. She had enjoyed great health her whole life up to that point. She'd been so proud that she wasn't on a single medication and that she felt great. But when she found a lump during a breast self-exam, things most definitely changed. I can imagine most people in their 80s who got a cancer diagnosis would probably think this was the beginning of the end, considering themselves lucky to have made it that long into life. But not Margaret; she looked right down the barrel of cancer and said, "You won't steal my spirit!" With the support of her loving family (I told you loved ones are critical!), she fought hard. She went through chemo, losing every last hair on her head, and she endured the miserable side effects that accompany aggressive cancer treatments. But perhaps the most significant strategy working in her favor was that of keeping a smile on her face. Her positive outlook, that sunny disposition, that ability to see the silver lining behind the dark cloud, was never once shaken. She told everyone that she'd been too healthy her whole life to just give up with cancer now. Her medical team was astounded at how well she did. I'm a firm believer that it was her attitude that got her through. Margaret is a cancer survivor, and she's still going strong.

Of course, I'm not naïve enough to say that if you just put a smile on your face you can survive any serious illness. But coupled with good medical care, a positive outlook can take your health and longevity to the next level. Here's how.

My 100 Happy, Healthy Years Prescription

Optimism for Optimal Health

If my story about Margaret wasn't powerful enough for you, here's the research to prove it. Sure, it's inherently obvious that being optimistic is good for your mental health. But did you know research is showing a connection between a positive attitude and good *physical* health? In fact, University of Michigan researchers did a study in which participants rated their levels of optimism. They discovered that for every point of reported optimism, the subjects' risk of having an acute stroke decreased by 9 percent. Furthermore, if you fall in the "glass half-full" category, you're more apt to safeguard your health by being physically active and making smart health choices across the board.

Write Your Way to Good Health

I'm a huge proponent of journaling. You could write about how your day went and accidentally learn something about yourself. It's amazing what happens when you just let it all out on paper or the computer screen: you'll de-stress by organizing your thoughts and you'll be able to see the big picture, and hopefully stop sweating the small stuff.

Plus, you guessed it, there's proof that it's even good for your health. A study at the University of Texas ultimately showed a connection between regular journaling and improved immunity. So, spend just

15 minutes a day journaling or even doing creative writing, and you're less likely to get sick.

What exactly do you write in a journal? That answer is as individual as you might imagine. Some ideas:

A record of your life; if so, try to write most days of the week.
Expressions of anger, in order to release it and or keep it from
   building.
Your life goals—and how you achieved them
New ideas you have generated
Thoughts, feelings, and observations
Your opinions

Spirituality

There is burgeoning research in the area of spirituality and how it affects our overall health and longevity. The effects of spirituality on the human body aren't as easily calculated as quantifiable factors such as cholesterol, blood pressure, and the like. Nevertheless, I can tell you what many of my patients have shared with me over the years, which is that spirituality, in various ways, has played a role in their sense of well-being. Now, I'm certainly not here to tell you what to believe. But it's at least worth mentioning that social and behavioral scientists are studying the relationship between health (both physical and mental) and spirituality. My humble opinion is that having some type of ideology that you follow, regardless of what that is, will likely give you a greater sense of calm, provide you with a better ability to tackle problems and stress as they arise, and potentially contribute to your good health as you go through life.

Grateful Heart = Healthy Body

In the day-to-day craziness of life, it's so easy to take a lot for granted. It's also easy to forget to just say "thank you." So you may be wondering what being thankful has to do with good health. Here's a look:

There was a 21-day study done on patients who had a neuromuscular disease. One group was told to think about all the things they were grateful for in their lives, and focus on them. The other group was asked to focus on other things in their lives, but nothing related to being grateful. Of the two groups, the one assigned to feel gratitude was more likely to get better and deeper sleep at night. They also experienced other health benefits, including lessened anxiety.

I find in my own practice that the happiest and healthiest patients tend to be the ones who appreciate even the little things in life. They don't focus on what they don't have, or what they are lacking. They live in the moment, grateful for every breath. Here's an idea: Thank someone today. Whether you want to thank your parents for raising you, or your high school English teacher for motivating you so long ago, or even your coffee barista for knowing just how to prepare your decaf cup of joe, take a moment and express your gratitude. I promise you'll like the results!

What I hope you take away from the information I've shared here is that every decision you make has some type of effect on the health of your whole body. Even if you've never eaten a candy bar and you work out religiously, you may not be as healthy as you think. Your lifestyle, your daily interaction, and your emotional health all play important roles in living 100 happy, healthy years. Savor every second.

CHAPTER 18

Cycle 4: 17 Day Plan

You've now completed the first three cycles of this plan and you've made a lot of progress over the past 51 days (but who's counting!). You've paid attention to each of your body systems, and they're likely returning the favor by performing at their peak. Take a moment and reflect on how much you've been able to change in this short period of time. You are making smarter food choices; movement and exercise have become a priority in your day regardless of how or where; you're drinking plenty of water; you're avoiding many of the habits that are harmful to your health; you're even doing Kegel exercises at the grocery store! All of these decisions, for which I commend you, are bringing about changes that you should feel proud of and be enjoying.

Perhaps the most exciting aspect is that you're doing work that will protect you in the long-term from all the uncomfortable, unhealthy, undesirable, and unattractive signs of aging. But believe it or not, there's more. The two chapters you just read, which focus on how you live your life and how you can avoid harmful environmental factors, play crucial roles in anti-aging. The great news is that you're already doing many of the things that will help your body fight off toxins. But just a few more adjustments can give you an overall sense of renewal and take your anti-aging benefits to a whole new level.

Some of the guidelines in this final cycle may seem strict, but there's a method to my madness. I'm trying to show you that these adjustments aren't as hard as you think, and they're so rewarding. For example, cutting out fast food completely for 17 days may seem tough, but you're on the verge of discovering how little you will actually miss it! It may also seem impossible to find time in your busy schedule to volunteer, but once you carve out the hours, you'll have a whole new appreciation of its value—not just to the world but also to your own well-being. You'll look back and wonder how you could ever *not* find the time for something so valuable, and hopefully make it a priority on an ongoing basis.

I developed this cycle with the goal of helping you learn something

257

priceless about yourself. It isn't about beating yourself up or feeling guilty. It's about renewing your faith in yourself (or discovering it for the first time) and appreciating your amazing ability to change, evolve, and grow.

Before Beginning Cycle 4

- Make a "grateful list" and keep it nearby.
  - Write down at least five things you're grateful for right now. You may include people you love, your job, your home, your health—anything that you are happy to have in your life but may sometimes take for granted.
  - Keep this list in your wallet or somewhere nearby during this cycle and refer to it at least once a day for a mental boost, especially if you're feeling pessimistic.
  - Add to your list anytime you see fit. Moments of gratitude may strike when you least expect them, and writing them down will only increase your appreciation.
- Update your cleaning supplies.
  - Take inventory of all your cleaning supplies and consider throwing out the ones with harsh chemicals. You'll probably notice when you look at their labels that some of them say they're hazardous to humans and domestic animals. These cleaners probably have chlorine or other potentially hazardous ingredients, especially for people with respiratory issues or allergies.
  - I know these supplies aren't cheap, so I'm not suggesting you throw them all out and start over. But consider throwing some away and replacing them with safer alternatives such as vinegar, baking soda, hydrogen peroxide, or nontoxic, environmentally safe and natural cleaning products.
  - Empty the products in your sink instead of simply tossing half-full bottles in the trash.
- Look into an indoor air purifier.

- Especially if you suffer from allergies, consider making the investment to purify the air in your home. You can buy an air purifier online or at home stores. I recommend ones with HEPA (high-efficiency particulate air) filters.

- Get your home tested for radon and carbon monoxide if:
  - You don't know when it was tested last.
  - You're buying a new home.
  - You recently renovated your home.
  - Your home hasn't been tested in the last two years.
  - You can also purchase testing kits online and do this yourself rather than hiring an expert to conduct the test. At-home kits range from $15 to $40, but make sure the one you buy is approved by the EPA.
  - If you have a carbon monoxide detector or alarm in your home, make sure it's functioning. Read the manufacturer's label to find out how to check for low batteries.

General Guidelines for Cycle 4

- When you're eating out at a restaurant:
  - If the restaurant has its menu posted online, check it beforehand to find the healthiest options and decide before you go what you will order. This not only gives you plenty of time to be sure you're picking one of the healthier options, but it will also help you stay strong when you're tempted by unhealthy options on the menu.
  - Avoid dishes that have these words in the menu listing: *battered, deep-fried, crusted, creamed* or *creamy, loaded, crispy, crunchy, scalloped, alfredo, à la mode, cheesy*. Think of them as unhealthy key words—they're the warning sign that you need to find something else to eat.
  - Look for these healthy key words, because the dishes will likely be lower in fat and calories: *steamed, sautéed, baked, boiled, poached, roasted, clear broth, puree*.

- Ask the waiter to prepare your food "dry," with no butter, lard, or oil. You'll cut way back on calories this way. You can even get the sauce on the side to try a few dips as opposed to having your meal be drenched in it.

- Remember that animal proteins prepared with high, dry heat (such as when they're fried or grilled) release more AGEs (advanced glycation end-products) than when they're prepared with wet heat (such as boiled or steamed). Ask your server to prepare your foods accordingly. Don't be embarrassed to ask for special preparation; most restaurants will accommodate you. You're the customer, so there's no harm in asking!

- Commit to giving up fast food during this cycle.

  - Every time you're tempted to pick up a greasy bag of fries and nuggets, drive to the closest grocery store and pick up a healthy snack instead.

  - Alternatively, use your craving as a time to meditate or get moving!

- Create a sleep schedule and stick with it.

  - Plan to get six to eight hours of sleep each night. Often, the easiest way to get into a pattern is to decide to go to bed and wake up at the same time each day. You were already doing this in Cycle 2, so it should be a simple habit to continue.

DAY 1

Morning: Look online or watch your local news to find out the outdoor air quality for your region. If the air quality is at unhealthy levels, make an effort to stay inside as much as possible.

Midday: Start doing research on where you might be able to volunteer at least once during this cycle. You might look into your local homeless shelters, animal shelters, food banks, and charitable organizations for inspiration, based on your passions. Make this a priority, even though your schedule is packed.

DAY 2

Morning: Check your local air quality.

Anytime: Hit up the grocery store.

- Bring the list of produce that I recommend purchasing organic. You can find this in Chapter 16. The idea is to stock your kitchen with the healthiest, most pesticide-free fruits and veggies.

- Buy a few glass storage containers to begin replacing the plastic ones you may have.

DAY 3

Morning: Check your local air quality. (You'll keep doing this every day, but by Day 4 it will feel second nature so you probably won't even need a reminder.)

Evening: Call a friend or family member and make plans to spend time together doing something you'll both enjoy. Spending time with friends can improve your immunity, lower your blood pressure, and improve your overall health. You may want to consider reconnecting with an old friend you haven't spoken to in a while; now's a great time to rekindle the friendship.

DAY 4

Anytime: Look into purchasing BPA-free plastic containers or water bottles today. Aside from buying new ones, you'll need to throw out any plastic containers you currently use.

DAY 5

Midday: If you haven't had your vitamin D levels checked recently, call your doctor and make an appointment to have them tested.

Evening: Make time to spend with your partner; connecting and experiencing intimacy can take effort, so make it a priority.

DAY 6

Evening: Start (or continue) a journal. Write in it every day or a few times a week. Focus on writing down your frustrations—and then letting them go. You'll be shocked at how freeing this can be!

DAY 7

Midday: Have you volunteered yet? Make it your goal to spend at least two hours volunteering before this cycle is over.

DAY 8

Morning: Check your local air quality.

Midday: How has your eating been? If you feel like it's hard to keep track of your food choices, start a food journal in which you record everything you eat, including the quantities. No cheating—if it goes in your mouth, it gets written down.

DAY 9

Morning: Check your local air quality.

Evening: Perform dry skin brushing. You can find out how on page 228.

DAY 10

Morning: Check your local air quality.

Midday: Make plans with several friends to get together in the next week.

DAY 11

Morning: Check your local air quality.

Anytime: Pay it forward today by making a donation, filling someone's expired parking meter with coins, purchasing coffee for the person in line behind you, letting someone who's rushed or with a child cut in front of you in line, holding the door open for someone, or just smiling at as many people as possible.

DAY 12

Morning: Check your local air quality.

Midday: Make an effort to say good morning to strangers, or "bless you" when someone sneezes, or "have a nice day" to someone.

DAY 13

Morning: Check your local air quality.

Evening: Make time to spend with your partner to connect and experience intimacy.

DAY 14

Morning: Check your local air quality.

Midday: If you haven't spent a couple of hours volunteering yet, make it a priority in the next two days.

DAY 15

Morning: Check your local air quality.

All day: Commit to ONLY eating fresh, whole foods. Don't eat anything today that is canned, boxed, or packaged.

- *Idea:* For breakfast, eat two hard-boiled eggs and an apple, then a spinach salad for lunch and a steamed veggie plate for dinner. Snack on nuts, seeds, and fruit throughout the day and only drink water.

DAY 16

Morning: Check your local air quality.

Anytime: Look at your air conditioner and air purifier filters and see if they need to be cleaned or replaced.

DAY 17

Morning: Check your local air quality.

Evening: Perform dry skin brushing.

Come on, I'm a doctor, so I know better than to think that your health is simply tied to saying "Good morning" to a passerby or to keeping a gratitude list. But I wouldn't be suggesting these things if I didn't believe they work. So many of us are living life in the fast lane, and our health is being compromised because of it. With this cycle, I hope I've put the power back in your hands to control your environment, replenish your spirit, and start enjoying life again. The goal here is not only to halt the aging process, but to make your 100 years healthy, happy, fulfilling years. I hope you're well on your way.

EPILOGUE

Let's face it: I can't stop you from getting older. I don't have a magical wand that stops the clock and keeps you looking and feeling 25 forever. Not that you even want that, because it would mean you wouldn't get to live your life, learn, grow, and evolve. After all, do you really want to be frozen in a sort of never-ending Groundhog Day? There is no magic bullet, no fountain of youth, and no mysterious method to arrest your body's deterioration. What I've just given you is something much better than all that. I've handed you the keys to unlock the hidden power within your own body; you've got the power to drastically slow the process of aging.

When you consider all of the advances in medical science, technology, and pharmaceuticals in the last five or so decades, people should really be living to be 150 years old! We have come so far in those areas, and the tools we doctors have at our disposal are simply incredible. I mean, we're doing robotic surgeries, for Pete's sake! Yet, on the whole, we aren't living nearly as long or as well as we should. What's gone wrong?

Often, the simplest answer is the correct one, so let's focus on getting back to basics. To me, it seems that society has collectively forgotten some fundamental truths about the human body. Let's not be overly reliant on medical tools, machines, surgeries, and pills to save us. Yes, I'm thrilled those things exist when we need them. But I fear too many people have started looking outside themselves for the solution, rather than realizing that excellent health really starts with the patient . . . that's you.

I sincerely hope you now understand that you don't have to just blindly accept all of the negative side effects of aging. Yes, you will get older. That's a good thing. But aging doesn't just happen to you. You control it. I want you to feel empowered to grab hold of the strategies I've laid out within the pages of this book and apply them right away. And I wish you the best that life has to offer on your way to 100 happy, healthy years. See you at 100!

APPENDIX

Breathing Techniques

"Breath of Fire"

Ask any yoga instructor to hold his or her breath as long as he or she can, and you'll be amazed. Why do yogis' lungs seem to have superhuman capacity? They know the secret to sending oxygen into the deepest regions of their lungs. Think your shallow chest breathing does that? Think again!

Here's how to practice an ancient breathing exercise called *Kapalabhati pranayama*, or "Breath of Fire." Sit up straight, in a comfortable position (preferably Indian style on the floor). Close your eyes and rest one hand gently on your stomach and your other hand on your thigh. Fully relax your stomach muscles. Start by sticking out your tongue and panting rapidly, like a dog. The breath is coming from your stomach, so your belly should be going in and out with each breath. Continue this for only a few seconds, then close your mouth and take the rapid breaths in and out through your nose. It should sound like really fast sniffing, but in a steady rhythm. Imagine you're blowing out a fire just under your nose!

Precaution: If you feel dizzy at all, stop Breath of Fire and go back to normal breathing. Check with your physician or skip this practice altogether if you've been diagnosed with high blood pressure, heart disease, or epilepsy. An alternative is sitting up straight and taking long, slow deep breaths in through the nose, out through the mouth.

Diaphragmatic Breathing Technique

Your diaphragm is a muscle across the bottom of your ribcage that helps you breathe. Singing coaches often advise their pupils to learn how to breathe using their diaphragm because it can help them not run out of air, especially when they're holding a particularly long note. I think everyone should work on this technique to help improve their overall breathing. Here's how to do it properly:

267

Sit upright in a chair and place your hand on your stomach so you can actually feel your muscles working. Slowly inhale through your nose while pushing your abdomen out as you breathe in. Hold your breath for a moment, and then exhale through your mouth while sucking in your tummy. This is a two-for-one, because it also works out your abdominal muscles!

Straw Breathing

Pinch your nose, and keep your lips sealed around the straw. Breathe for one minute. If you feel dizzy, stop.

Laughter Yoga

Laughter Yoga is the combination of yogic breathing and unconditional laughter. The focus is to continuously laugh throughout the exercises. Your body can't tell the difference between forced and real laughter, so you're getting the same benefits as if you were laughing at your favorite joke! To do this, sit Indian style on the floor. This is a "fake it till you make it" type of exercise, so begin by faking laughter. Once you fake it for a few seconds, you'll probably start cracking up at yourself and before you know it, you'll hardly be able to stop laughing. For even more fun, try doing this with a friend or partner. You'll feel silly at first, but I promise it's worth it.

Cardiovascular Exercises

Wall Sits

Stand with your back against a wall. Begin to slide your upper body down the wall as you bend your knees, as if you are sitting on a chair. Your knees should be at a 90-degree angle, right above your heels. Your arms should be down by your sides, palms against the wall. If you put your hands on your legs, you are cheating. Hold this for 30 to 60 seconds, and make sure to keep your abs contracted!

Squats

Stand with your legs about shoulder-width apart. Keeping your back straight, lower your hips until your thighs are parallel to the floor. Make sure your body weight is on the back of your heels. Slowly stand back up to complete one squat.

Jumping Jacks

Start by standing with legs together, arms down by your sides. Jump so that your feet land about shoulder-width apart. At the same time, bring your arms upward, so your hands reach above your head. Jump again, this time bringing your legs back together while simultaneously bringing your arms downward back to your sides. Repeat. The faster you do this, the higher your heart rate will climb.

Squat Jacks

These are like jumping jacks but in a squat position, for more intense engagement of your quadriceps (thigh muscles). Stand with your feet shoulder-width apart, put your hands behind your head (optional for more of a challenge), and squat (back straight, lower your hips until your thighs are parallel to the floor), then jump up and land in your beginning squat position. The tendency is to straighten your legs, so fight to keep the bend in your knees.

Lunges

Stand with your feet just slightly apart. Take a big step forward with your right foot, lowering your body toward the ground by bending your right knee at a 90-degree angle. Make sure your knee doesn't extend past your toe. Remember to keep your back leg straight and avoid any wobbling by contracting your abs! It will help to keep your hands on your hips while bending your knee. Return to your standing position and repeat this motion with your opposite foot.

Explosive Jump Lunges

Get into lunge stance. Powerfully jump upward, switching legs midair so that your left foot is in front, leading the lunge when you land. Note—this is an advanced exercise and you shouldn't do it until you feel completely ready.

Shadowboxing

Stand with knees slightly bent. Make a fist and begin throwing jabs and cross punches, alternating arms. Keep your arms slightly bent at all times and be careful not to overextend your elbows.

Chair Squats

While standing, slowly squat down over a chair until your butt hovers just above the seat, and then go back up. Keep your chest up and focus your eyes forward so you don't lean over too much and make this too easy.

Stretches

Standing Chest Expansion

Stand up straight, keeping your arms down at your sides. Bring your arms behind you and interlace fingers, keeping the arms straight. Slowly start bending backward while looking up, pulling your chest wide. You should feel the stretch across your chest. Take two deep breaths.

Cobra Stretches

Lie facedown on your stomach. Keep your hands by your shoulders (as though you're going to do a push-up) and begin to push your torso up as far as you can, straightening your arms. Tip your head back and look at the ceiling as you stretch out your abdominal wall and chest. Take three deep breaths, in and out. *Important:* You shouldn't feel pain, just a nice, deep stretch!

Cat/Cow Stretches

Get on your hands and knees. Keep your hands directly under your shoulders. If the floor is too hard for your knees, put a towel or small pillow underneath them. Take a deep breath in as you arch your back, and then breathe out as you curve it. This should be a slow and methodical movement.

Butt Kickers

Stand up, bend one knee, and lift your heel as close to your butt as possible. Repeat on the other side. This stretches your quadriceps. You can do this slowly as a stretch or fast for a cardio workout.

Diagonal Neck Stretch

Turn your head slightly. Look down, as if gazing into your pocket. Hold and repeat on each side.

Ankle Circles

In a seated position, stetch your legs out in front of you. Point your toes and make a circle with your big toe. Go 10 times clockwise, and 10 times counterclockwise.

Executive Stretch

While seated, lock your hands behind your head. Bring your elbows back as far as possible. Inhale deeply during the stretch.

Arm Circles

When standing, make large windmill motions with your arms. You can rotate arms one at a time, in alternating motions, or simultaneously. Switch it up by circling arms both forward and backward. Do this slowly at first, and then you can pick up some speed.

High-Sodium Foods

You may be keeping a close eye on the fat and calorie content of what you're eating, but are you keeping track of the amount of sodium in those foods? The American Medical Association says 150,000 lives could be saved each year if Americans just cut out half of their salt intake! It's recommended that the average person consume no more than 2,300 milligrams per day, but Americans are actually averaging 4,000 to 5,000 milligrams per day. Here's how to control your intake:

How to Determine "High in Sodium"

- Avoid products with more than 200 milligrams of sodium per serving. Remember to check closely for serving size, taking into consideration how many servings you will realistically eat.
- Avoid foods that have more milligrams of sodium in them than number of calories.

* Know your labels.

    * **Sodium-free or salt-free.** Each serving will have less than five milligrams of sodium.

    * **Very low sodium.** Each serving will have 35 milligrams of sodium or less.

    * **Low sodium.** Each serving will have 140 milligrams of sodium or less.

    * **Reduced or less sodium.** The product contains at least 25 percent less sodium than the regular version. (But watch out! The original version may have had a very high amount of sodium, so this product could still have a higher amount than recommended.)

    * **Lite or light in sodium.** The sodium content has been reduced by at least 50 percent from the regular version. (Keep in mind how much sodium the original product has.)

    * **Unsalted or no salt added.** No salt is added during the processing of a food that normally contains salt. (Just because no salt was added during processing doesn't make this food a safe bet! Some of the ingredients may be high in sodium.)

Unexpected High-Sodium Culprits

Salsa—1 cup—1,554 mg
Baking soda—1 tsp—1,259 mg (remember—many recipes call for baking soda)
Potato chips—one 8-ounce bag—1,090 mg
Hummus—1 cup—932 mg
Low-fat cottage cheese (1% milk)—1 cup—918 mg
Pasta with tomato sauce, no meat—1 cup—647 mg
Steak sauce (tomato based)—2 tbsp—560 mg
Soy sauce—1 tbsp—1,000 mg
Marinara sauce—½ cup—553 mg
Oat bran bagel—4-inch diameter—532 mg
Pita bread—one (6-inch diameter)—340 mg
Dill pickles—large (4 inches): 1,181 mg / small: 324 mg
Commercial Italian salad dressing—2 tbsp—300 mg
Microwave popcorn—1 ounce—300 mg
Ketchup—one packet—100 mg

Lower-Sodium Alternatives:

* Fresh vegetables instead of canned

* Homemade soups instead of canned

* Pepper, garlic powder, or parsley

* Fresh lemons

Sodium Tips When Eating Out

- Ask to have your entree prepared without extra salt.
- Portion sizes at restaurants are usually very large. Put half of your dish in a to-go box, and enjoy it as a separate meal.

Your Important Heart Measurements

How to Take Resting Heart Rate

- Your pulse is the rate at which your heart beats. Your pulse is usually called your heart rate, which is the number of times your heart beats each minute (bpm).
  - To check your pulse, find the large vein on the wrist that lies in line with the thumb. Do not use your thumb, because it has its own pulse that you may feel.
  - Count the beats for 30 seconds, and then multiply that number by two to get the number of beats per minute.

Cardio Zone

- Do the math
  - For moderate-intensity physical activity, a person's target heart rate should be 60 to 80 percent of his or her maximum heart rate.
  - Estimate your maximum heart rate by subtracting your age from 220.
  - Find out what your target heart rate should be by multiplying your bpm by .5 and .7.
  - If your bpm falls in between those two numbers, you are in the target heart rate zone!
  - **Take the talk test:** While you are doing cardio, say a sentence out loud. If you can't finish the sentence easily because you're too winded, you are overdoing it. If you can spit out the sentence with ease, step up your workout!

Push and Pull Exercises

Push Exercises

Exercises that involve pushing, challenging your triceps, chest, and shoulders.

- **Push-ups**—On the floor with legs straight out behind you, form a straight board with your body. You will be resting on your hands and toes. Keep your elbows extended and hands shoulder-width apart. Slowly lower your body toward the floor by bending your elbows until your chest is parallel to the ground. Push your body back up by re-extending your elbows.

- **T Push-ups**—Start in normal push-up formation. As you raise your body into the "up" position, twist your body by rotating your hips open so that all of your weight is on one hand and the other arm is pointing toward the sky. Go back down to starting position. Alternate arms every time you lift your body up.

- **Wall Push-ups**—Stand facing a wall at arm's length. Put your hands flat on the wall and slowly bend your elbows so you are leaning into the wall. Push against the wall until your elbows are straight, keeping hands on wall. To make the workout more difficult, stand even farther from the wall.

- **Triceps Dip**—Sit on a chair with your legs together, stretched straight out in front of you. Grip your hands on the edge of the seat and scoot forward, so your arms are holding your body up. Straighten your arms with a little bend to ensure you're working your triceps and not hurting your elbow joints. Slowly lower your body by bending your elbows until your butt is almost touching the ground. Lift your body up and repeat.

Pull Exercises

Pulling exercises target the upper back, the back of the shoulders, and the biceps.

- **Chin-ups**—Place your hands shoulder-width apart on a sturdy horizontal bar, fingers facing toward you. Pull yourself upward until your chin is just over the bar. Slowly lower yourself back down and repeat.

- **Bicep Curls**—Hold a five-to-10-pound weight in each hand. Start with your arms straight down at your sides. Keep your elbows squeezed tightly against your hips. Raise your arms, bending at the elbow, lifting the weights all the way. Slowly lower the weights back down to your sides. Focus on not letting your elbows move while you raise and lower arms.

- **Shrugs**—While standing, hold two dumbbells of equal weight at your sides. Elevate and pull your shoulders up and down. Make sure to keep your head straight.

* **Rowing Machine**—While sitting on the machine's seat, reach forward and grab the bar handle, pulling back until the chain is taut. Slowly bend your knees, allowing your body to slide forward. Extend your legs to push your body back out. Make sure not to lean forward and to keep your back flat when sliding back and forth.

Leg Exercises

Improve strength in your upper and lower legs with the following exercises.

Couch Leg Extensions

Use your couch for this exercise. Rest your hands on the arm of the couch, holding your body up in plank position. Make sure your legs are extended straight out behind you. Lift one leg as high as you can, then slowly return it to the floor. Repeat with the same leg for one minute and then switch to the opposite leg.

Side Leg Lifts

Lie on your side with your lower leg bent and upper leg straight. Slowly lift the upper leg into the air before lowering it back down. Repeat for one minute and then flip over, switching to the opposite leg. It's important to remember to keep your hips parallel with your shoulders.

Climbing Stairs

Climb up and down stairs. Add variety to this workout by skipping every other stair.

Jump Squats

Get in the squat position: legs shoulder-width apart and knees at a 90-degree angle, keeping your back straight. Jump high into the air, extending your legs. As you come back down, land softly, reassuming squat position.

Calf Raises

Stand hip-width apart, feet flat on the ground. Using your calf muscles, raise up on your toes, balancing your body weight on the balls of your feet. Hold briefly before slowly returning your feet flat to the floor.

Core Exercises

Focus on the core muscles of the abdomen and back to preserve mobility and protect your back muscles.

Sit-ups

Lie on your back, knees bent, feet flat on the ground. Cross your arms over your chest. Use your abs to pull your shoulders and upper body toward your knees. Once you've pulled your body all the way up into a sitting position, slowly lower your torso back to the floor, flexing your abs as you go.

Crunches

Crunches are different from sit-ups because with crunches, you *don't* want to lift your back fully off the ground, and they are much shorter movements. Get in a sit-up position with knees bent, feet flat on the floor. Raise your shoulders toward your knees and lower your back toward the ground without letting your head touch the floor.

Plank

Get into a push-up position, but hold yourself up by the forearms rather than the hands. Hold your body flat like a board. Do not sag or arch your back.

Side Twists

Sit on the floor and cross your arms over your chest. Lean back so your upper body makes a 45-degree angle to the floor. Rotate your torso to the right while bringing your right knee toward your chest. Your left elbow should be touching your right knee. Now rotate your torso to the left as you bring your left knee toward your chest.

Bicycles

Lie face up on the floor and lightly place your hands behind your head. Bring your knees in to your chest and lift your shoulder blades off the floor. Rotate your torso to the left, bringing your right elbow toward your left knee as you straighten the other leg. Rotate in the opposite direction, bringing in the right knee and extending the left, so now your left elbow is touching your right knee. The trick to this exercise is mimicking a "pedaling" motion with your legs.

Balance Exercises

Heel-Toe Walk

Walk heel to toe along an imaginary straight line while focusing your gaze on something in front of you; do not look at your feet. Do this exercise for one minute.

Stork Stance

While standing, lift one leg off the ground and position the foot against the inside of the standing knee. To help with balance, fix your eyes on something in front of you. Engage your core muscles to maintain balance. Try closing your eyes. Hold each side for 30 seconds.

Weight Shifts

Stand with feet hip-width apart. Slowly lift one leg sideways so your foot is off the floor as you shift your weight to the opposite side. Hold, then switch legs.

Ball Around Back

Stand on one leg. Take a ball and circle it behind your back and around your waist while keeping your balance. Also try with your eyes closed.

Sit to Stand

Sit on the edge of a chair. Without using your hands, stand up while keeping your balance. Slowly lower yourself back to sitting.

Tips for Making Water Tasty

Add Natural Flavor

* Get a big jug, fill it with pure water, chop up a few cucumbers, and let them soak for a refreshing crispness.
* Drop a few squeezes of lemon in your water for a boost of citrus.
* Freeze your favorite fruits, such as strawberries or blueberries, and add them as ice cubes to your next glass of water.
* Add a few drops of peppermint extract and make your own mint water.
* Add ginger for some zing in your water.

Add Some Excitement

* Get all-natural, sugar-free seltzer as a bubbly twist on plain water.

Turn Water into Tea

* Try a fruit-flavored herbal tea. There are some great caffeine-free flavors such as peach, blueberry, and apple.

Ideas for Veggie Haters

Hide them in spaghetti sauce

Zucchini, onion, puréed carrots, spinach, bell pepper, and celery will each give your sauce a punch of vitamins.

Snack on them with fruit

Cut up cucumbers and combine them with watermelon chunks. Include chopped mint leaves for a great snack.

Go green with your smoothie

Take your favorite fruit smoothie mix and toss in a couple of cups of frozen spinach or fresh basil for a filling, healthy drink.

- Banana Basil Blend: Blend two bananas, 10 basil leaves (fresh is better), one tablespoon honey, ¼ cup cranberry juice, and a few cubes of ice.
- Spinach Super Smoothie: Blend one handful of fresh spinach, one cup vanilla low-fat yogurt, ½ cup cranberry juice, ½ cup strawberries (fresh or frozen), ½ cup blueberries, one banana (fresh or frozen), and a few cubes of ice.

Mix up your ground meat

Finely diced veggies are a good addition to any ground beef, chicken, or turkey dish. Meat loaf, chili, hamburgers, and meatballs could all be spruced up with some carrots, peppers, onions, or zucchini.

Refine your wraps

Make a healthy Mexican-inspired wrap by mashing up nutritious black beans and spreading them on a tortilla with low-fat cheese and some quinoa. You can also add finely grated peppers or broccoli to any chicken wrap.

Sub in the spinach

Boost the vitamins in your sub by subbing in spinach to replace your shredded lettuce. Try your sub with a handful of sprouts, too!

Resources to Help You Quit Smoking

Cleveland Clinic Program

At this treatment program you'll meet with a specialist to go over your medical history and your history of tobacco use. Get a treatment plan specific to your needs, with the option of web-based, individual, or group counseling. This program also offers nontraditional strategies such as hypnosis and acupuncture. All sessions are outpatient and last about 20 to 40 minutes (http://my.clevelandclinic.org/tobacco/default.aspx).

American Cancer Society

This online program provides general information on the harms of smoking, current types of nicotine replacement therapies, and the latest smoking statistics. You can also learn the difference between nicotine's mental and physical addiction (http://www.cancer.org/Healthy/StayAwayfromTobacco/GuidetoQuittingSmoking/).

American Lung Association

The "Freedom from Smoking" group clinic includes eight sessions and a step-by-step guide to quitting. They help smokers take control over their behavior by encouraging participants to work in groups, as well as on their own. There is even an online version of the program, and you can test it out for free (http://www.lung .org/stop-smoking/how-to-quit/).

Mayo Clinic

The Mayo Clinic Nicotine Dependence Center focuses on support and motivation and helps you develop an individualized plan, often consisting of a combination of counseling and medication. They have programs supervised by doctors, and they even have an eight-day residential treatment program (http://www.mayoclinic.org/ stop-smoking/).

American Heart Association

On their website, you will learn how to fight the cigarette urges, avoid gaining weight once you quit, and track your personal heart health. There is also a heart attack risk assessment tool (http://www.heart.org/HEARTORG/GettingHealthy/ QuitSmoking/Quit-Smoking_UCM_001085_SubHomePage.jsp).

National Cancer Institute

This program allows you to get real-time help without leaving your home. Use Live-Help, their confidential instant messaging service, to chat with information specialists about cancer, clinical trials, and quitting smoking. Get 24-hour support by signing up for their text messaging service, SmokefreeTXT, which is free and designed to send you periodic reminders and encouragement, keeping you on track (http://www.smokefree.gov/).

UCLA Addiction Medicine and Smoking Cessation Program

Specializing in treating patients who have tried to quit smoking before, UCLA Smoking Cessation Program will utilize outpatient therapy and approved medications to help you quit for good (http://www.uclahealth.org/body.cfm?id=453& action=detail&limit_department=14&limit_division=0&limit_program=5391&CFID =69815709&CFTOKEN=30286044).

WebMD

On their website, you will learn your cigarette triggers, develop a strategy to quit, and once you do, receive help to stay on track. They support you with expert blogs, articles, and community support groups (http://www.webmd.com/smoking -cessation/default.htm).

Cedars-Sinai Smoking Cessation Program

This program provides personal one-on-one therapy sessions with a clinical pharmacist, a personalized plan to help you quit, advice on how to curb cravings and control urges, and carbon monoxide monitoring of your lungs on every visit. You can take single sessions at $25 per visit (http://www.cedars-sinai.edu/Patients/ Physicians/Cedars-Sinai-Medical-Group/Treatments-and-Programs/Smoking -Cessation-Program.aspx).

CDC

The Centers for Disease Control's Office on Smoking and Health is dedicated to reducing deaths and disease caused by tobacco use or exposure to secondhand smoke. On their website, you can read success stories and tips from former smokers and connect with other smokers through social media (http://www.cdc.gov/ tobacco/quit_smoking/).

RESOURCES

Introduction

Costa, P. T., and R. R. McCrae. 1980. Somatic complaints in males as a function of age and neuroticism: A longitudinal analysis. *Journal of Behavioral Medicine* 3: 245–57.

Chapter 1: Five Factors of Aging

Abramson, J. L., and V. Vaccarino. 2002. Relationship between physical activity and inflammation among apparently healthy middle-aged and older US adults. *Archives of Internal Medicine* 162(11): 1286–92.

Heilbronn, L. K., et al. 2006. Effect of 6-month calorie restriction on biomarkers of longevity, metabolic adaptation, and oxidative stress in overweight individuals: A randomized controlled trial. *Journal of the American Medical Association* 295(13): 1539–48.

Toth, M. J., A. Tchernof, et al. 2000. Regulation of protein metabolism in middle-aged, premenopausal women: Roles of adiposity and estradiol. *Journal of Clinical Endocrinology & Metabolism* 85(4): 1382–87.

Verhoef, P., et al. 2002. Contribution of caffeine to the homocysteine-raising effect of coffee: A randomized controlled trial in humans. *American Journal of Clinical Nutrition* 76 (6): 1244–48.

Yunsheng, M., et al. 2006. Association between dietary fiber and serum C-reactive protein. *The American Journal of Clinical Nutrition* 83 (4): 760–66.

Chapter 2: Build Your Anti-Aging Base

Rush University Medical Center, Rush Nutrition and Wellness Center. What is a healthy weight? http://www.rush.edu/rumc/page-1108048103230.html.

Chapter 3: The Heart of the Matter

American Heart Association. June 2011. About arrhythmia. http://www.heart.org/
    HEARTORG/Conditions/Arrhythmia/AboutArrhythmia/About-Arrhyth
    mia_UCM_002010_Article.jsp.

Jankord, R., and B. Jemiolo. 2004. Influence of physical activity on serum IL-6 and
    IL-10 levels in healthy older men. *Medicine and Science in Sports and Exer-
    cise* 36(6): 960–64.

McCrory, M. A., et al. 1999. Dietary variety within food groups: Association with
    energy intake and body fatness in men and women. *American Journal of
    Clinical Nutrition* 69(3): 440–47.

Ridker, P. M., et al. 2005. C-reactive protein levels and outcomes after statin therapy.
    New England Journal of Medicine 352: 20–28.

Ridker, P. M., et al. 1998. Prospective study of C-reactive protein and the risk of
    future cardiovascular events among apparently healthy women. *American
    Heart Association*. Circulation. 98: 731–33.

Roger, V. L., et al., 2012. Heart disease and stroke statistics update. A report from the
    American Heart Association. *American Heart Association Statistical Update*.
    Circulation. 125: e2–e22.

Sachdeva, A., et al. 2009. Lipid levels in patients hospitalized with coronary artery
    disease: An analysis of 136,905 hospitalizations in Get with the Guide-
    lines. *American Heart Journal* 157(1): 111–17.

Thornton, S. N. 2010. Thirst and hydration: Physiology and consequences of dys-
    function. *Physiology and Behavior* 100(1): 15–21.

U.S. Department of Agriculture and U.S. Department of Health and Human Services.
    2010. Dietary guidelines for Americans 2010. http://health.gov/dietary
    guidelines/dga2010/dietaryguidelines2010.pdf (accessed June 4, 2012).

U.S. Department of Agriculture 2012. Agriculture Research Service, National Agricul-
    ture Library. National Nutrient Database for Standard Reference.

Zhang, X., et al. 2011. Cruciferous vegetable consumption is associated with a
    reduced risk of total and cardiovascular disease mortality. *American Journal
    of Clinical Nutrition* 94(1): 240–24.

Chapter 4: Breathe Easy

American Lung Association. 2011. Join us in the fight for air. http://www.lung.org/
    associations/charters/upper-midwest/about-us/2011-alaum-case-state
    ment.pdf.

Aoshiba, K., and A. Nagai. 2003. Oxidative stress, cell death, and other damage to
    alveolar epithelial cells induced by cigarette smoke. *Tobacco Induced Dis-
    eases* 1.3: 219–26. Accessed June 4, 2012. http://www.ncbi.nlm.nih.gov/
    pubmed/19570263.

Asthma and Allergy Foundation of America. 2005. Asthma overview. http://www.aafa.org/display.cfm?id=8&cont=5.

Baik, H. W., and R. M. Russell. 1999. Vitamin B12 deficiency in the elderly. *Annual Review of Nutrition* 19: 357–77.

Centers for Disease Control and Prevention. 2011. Asthma in the US, Growing every year. *CDC Vital Signs* (May 2011).

Knekt, P., et al. 2002. Flavonoid intake and risk of chronic diseases. *American Journal of Clinical Nutrition* 76(3): 560–68.

Leboeuf-Yde, C., et al. 2005. Self-reported nonmusculoskeletal responses to chiropractic intervention: A multination survey. *Journal of Manipulative and Physiological Therapeutics* 28(5): 294–302; discussion 365–56.

Le Marchand, L., et al. 2000. Intake of flavonoids and lung cancer. *Journal of the National Cancer Institute* 92(2): 154–60.

Linseisen, J., et al. 2007. Fruit and vegetable consumption and lung cancer risk: Updated information from the European Prospective Investigation into Cancer and Nutrition (EPIC). *International Journal of Cancer* 121(5): 1103–14.

Noble, J. M., et al., 2009. Periodontitis is associated with cognitive impairment among older adults: analysis of NHANES-III. *Journal of Neurology, Neurosurgery & Psychiatry* 80(11): 1206–1211. http://www.ncbi.nlm.nih.gov/pmc/articles/PMC3073380/.

Oh, R. C., and D. Brown. 2003. Vitamin B12 deficiency. *American Family Physician* 67(5): 979–86.

Pennypacker, L. C., et al. 1992. High prevalence of cobalamin deficiency in elderly outpatients. *Journal of the American Geriatrics Society* 40: 1197–204.

Rush University Medical Center. Breathe easier: tips for keeping your lungs healthy. http://www.rush.edu/rumc/page-1282236970456.html. May 21, 2012.

Schünemann, H.J., et al. 2001. The relation of serum levels of antioxidant vitamins C and E, retinol and carotenoids with pulmonary function in the general population. *American Journal of Respiratory and Critical Care Medicine* 163(5): 1246–55.

Schwartz, A. G., 2012. Genetic epidemiology of cigarette smoke-induced lung disease. *Proceedings of the American Thoracic Society* 9(2): 22–26.

Semba, R. D., et al., 2012. Serum carotenoids and pulmonary function in older community-dwelling women. *Journal of Nutrition, Health, & Aging* 16(4): 291–96.

Sepper, R., et al. 2012. Mucin5B expression by lung alveolar macrophages is increased in long-term smokers. *Journal of Leukocyte Biology* (May 16).

Studenski, S., et al. 2011. Gait speed and survival in older adults. *Journal of the American Medical Association* 305(1): 50–58.

U.S. Department of Agriculture. 2012. Agriculture Research Service, National Agriculture Library. National Nutrient Database for Standard Reference.

World Health Organization. 2011. Chronic obstructive pulmonary disease (COPD). Fact Sheet N°315. http://www.who.int/mediacentre/factsheets/fs315/en/index.html.

Chapter 5: Brainpower

Akbaraly, T. N., et al. 2007. Plasma selenium over time and cognitive decline in the elderly. *Epidemiology* 18(1): 52–58.

Ball, K., et al. 2002. Effects of cognitive training interventions with older adults. A randomized controlled trial. *Journal of the American Medical Association* 288(18): 2271–81.

Caprio, T. V., and Williams, T. F. 2007. Comprehensive geriatric assessment. *Practice of Geriatrics*, 4th ed., chap 4.

Chung, C. S., and L. R. Caplan. 2007. Stroke and other neurovascular disorders. In: Goetz, C. G., ed. *Textbook of Clinical Neurology*, 3rd ed. Philadelphia: Saunders Elsevier, chap. 45.

Durga, J., et al., 2005. Effect of lowering of homocysteine levels on inflammatory markers. A randomized controlled trial. *Archives of Internal Medicine* 165(12): 1388–94.

Ghosh, D., M. K. Mishra, S. Das, D. K. Kaushik, and A. Basu. 2009. Tobacco carcinogen induces microglial activation and subsequent neuronal damage. *Journal of Neurochemistry* 110: 1070–81.

Hile, E. S., and S. A. Studenski. 2007. Instability and falls. In: Duthie E. H., P. R. Katz, and M. L. Malone, eds., *Practice of Geriatrics*, 4th ed., chap. 17.

Ho, A. J., C. A. Raji, J. T. Becker, et al. 2010. Obesity is linked with lower brain volume in 700 AD and MCI patients. *Neurobiology of Aging* 31(8): 1326–39.

Kelkel, M., et al. 2010. Potential of the dietary antioxidants resveratrol and curcumin in prevention and treatment of hematologic malignancies. *Molecules.* 15(10): 7035–74.

Lambourne, K. 2006. The relationship between working memory capacity and physical activity rates in young adults. *Journal of Sports Science and Medicine* 5: 149–53.

Lançon, A., et al. 2012. Control of microRNA expression as a new way for resveratrol to deliver its beneficial effects. *Journal of Agriculture and Food Chemistry* (May).

Luders, E., et al. 2011. Enhanced brain connectivity in long-term meditation practitioners. *NeuroImage* 57(4): 1308–16.

Masoumi, A., et al., 2009. 1alpha,25-dihydroxyvitamin D3 interacts with curcuminoids to stimulate amyloid-beta clearance by macrophages of Alzheimer's disease patients. *Journal of Alzheimer's Disease* 17(3): 703–17.

Milara, J., and J. Cortijo. 2012. Tobacco, inflammation, and respiratory tract cancer. *Current Pharmaceutical Design.* Accessed June 4, 2012. http://www.ncbi.nlm.nih.gov/pubmed/22632749.

Oude Griep, L. M., et al. 2011. Colors of fruit and vegetables and 10-year incidence of stroke. *Stroke: A Journal of Cerebral Circulation*. 42(11): 3190–95.

Pierluigi, Q., et al. 2004. Homocysteine, folate, and vitamin B-12 in mild cognitive impairment, Alzheimer disease, and vascular dementia. *American Journal of Clinical Nutrition* 80(1): 114–22.

Seeman, T. E., et al. 2011. Histories of social engagement and adult cognition: Midlife in the U.S. study. *Journals of Gerontology, Series B, Psychological Sciences and Social Sciences* 66(Suppl. 1): 141–52.

Small, G. W., et al. 2009. Your brain on Google: Patterns of cerebral activation during internet searching. *American Journal of Geriatric Psychiatry* 17(2): 116–26.

Stewart, R., et al. 2008. Oral health and cognitive function in the Third National Health and Nutrition Examination Survey (NHANES III) Psychosomatic Medicine. *Journal of Biobehavioral Medicine* 70(8): 936–41.

U.S. Department of Agriculture. 2012. *Agriculture Research Service, National Agriculture Library. National Nutrient Database for Standard Reference*. Maryland, Nutrient Data Laboratory.

U.S. National Library of Medicine and National Institutes of Health. 2010. Aging changes in the senses. http://www.nlm.nih.gov/medlineplus/ency/article/004013.htm.

Zandi, P. P., et al. 2004. Reduced risk of Alzheimer disease in users of antioxidant vitamin supplements: The Cache County Study. *Archives of Neurology*. 61(1): 82–88.

Chapter 7: Your Body's Guard

Algra, A., et al. 2012. Effects of regular aspirin on long-term cancer incidence and metastasis: A systematic comparison of evidence from observational studies versus randomised trials. *Lancet Oncology* 13(5): 518–27.

Arthur, J., et al. 2003. Selenium in the immune system. *Journal of Nutrition* 133(5): 14575–595.

Bennett, M. P., et al. 2003. The effect of mirthful laughter on stress and natural killer cell activity. *Alternative Therapies in Health and Medicine* 9(2): 38–45.

Choi, M. 2009. The not-so-sweet side of fructose. *Journal of the American Society of Nephrology* 20(3): 457–59.

Cole, S., et al. 2008. Sleep loss activates cellular inflammatory signaling. *Biological Psychiatry* 64(6): 538–40.

Edlund, M. 2012. Getting healthy now. Regenerating yourself—using the right information. *Psychology Today* (May 17). http://www.psychologytoday.com/blog/getting-healthy-now/201205/regenerating-yourself-using-the-right-information?page=2.

Geisler, C., et al. 2010. Vitamin D controls T cell antigen receptor signaling and activation of human T cells. *Nature Immunology* 11: 344–49.

Johnson, R., et al. 2010. The Effect of Fructose on Renal Biology and Disease. *Journal of the American Society of Nephrology* 21(12): 2036–39.

Miller, M., and W. Fry, 2009. The effect of mirthful laughter on the human cardiovascular system. *Medical Hypotheses* 73(5): 636.

Miller, M., et al. 2009. University of Maryland School of Medicine study shows laughter helps blood vessels function better.

Office of Dietary Supplements: National Institutes of Health. Dietary supplement fact sheet: Selenium. http://ods.od.nih.gov/factsheets/SeleniumHealth Professional/.

Sugawara J., et al. 2010. Effect of mirthful laughter on vascular function. *American Journal of Cardiology* 106(6): 856–59.

Chapter 8: Listen to Your Gut

American Cancer Society. 2011. Colorectal cancer. http://www.cancer.org/Cancer/ColonandRectumCancer/DetailedGuide/colorectl-cancer-key-statistics.

American Cancer Society. 2011. Stomach cancer. http://www.cancer.org/Cancer/StomachCancer/DetailedGuide/stomach-cancerprevention.

American Cancer Society. 2011. What is small intestine cancer. http://www.cancer.org/Cancer/SmallIntestineCancer/DetailedGuide/smallintestine-cancer-what-is-small-intestine-cancer.

American Cancer Society. 2012. Stomach cancer overview. http://www.cancer.org/Cancer/StomachCancer/OverviewGuide/stomach-canceroverview-what-causes.

American College of Gastroenterology. Acid reflux. http://patients.gi.org/topics/acid-reflux/.

American College of Gastroenterology. 2010. Rectal problems. http://www.acg.gi.org/patients/women/rectal.asp.

Blot, W. J., et al. 1993. Nutrition intervention trials in Linxian, China: Supplementation with specific vitamin/mineral combinations, cancer incidence, and disease specific mortality in the general population. *Journal of the National Cancer Institute* 85(18): 1483–92.

Bogardus, S. T. 2006. What do we know about diverticular disease? A brief overview. *Journal of Clinical Gastroenterology* 40: S108–S11.

Centers for Disease Control and Prevention. 2006. Helicobacter pylori and peptic ulcer disease. The key to cure. http://www.cdc.gov/ulcer/keytocure.htm.

Chao, A., et al. 2002. Cigarette smoking, use of other tobacco products and stomach cancer mortality in US adults: The Cancer Prevention Study II. *International Journal of Cancer* 101(4): 380–89.

Hunt, R. H. 1996. *Helicobacter pylori*: From theory to practice. Proceedings of a symposium. *American Journal of Medicine* 100(5A): supplement.

Hunt, R. H., and A. B. R. Thompson. 1998. Canadian Helicobacter pylori Consensus Conference. *Canadian Journal of Gastroenterology* 12(1): 31–41.

Jacobs, E. J., et al. 2002. Vitamin C, vitamin E, and multivitamin supplement use and stomach cancer mortality in the Cancer Prevention Study II cohort. *Cancer Epidemiology, Biomarkers, & Prevention* 11(1): 35–41.

Jenab, M., et al. 2010. Association between pre-diagnostic circulation vitamin D concentration and risk of colorectal cancer in European populations: A nested case-control study. *BMJ* 340: b5500.

Johns Hopkins Health Alerts. October 2011. Diverticulosis and diverticulitis. http://www.johnshopkinshealthalerts.com/symptoms_remedies/diverticular_disorders/90-1.html.

Johns Hopkins Medicine Health Alerts. October 2011. Digestive disorders. http://www.johnshopkinshealthalerts.com/alerts_index/digestive_health/19-1.html.

Koizumi, Y. 2004. Cigarette smoking and the risk of gastric cancer: A pooled analysis of two prospective studies in Japan. *International Journal of Cancer* 112(6): 1049–55.

Mayo Clinic. Small bowel cancer. http://www.mayoclinic.org/small-bowel-cancer/.

National Cancer Institute. 2008. Garlic and cancer prevention. 2008. http://www.cancer.gov/cancertopics/factsheet/prevention/garlicand-cancer-prevention.

National Institute of Diabetes and Digestive and Kidney Disease, National Institutes of Health. 2008. Diverticulosis and diverticulitis. Publication No. 08–1163.

National Institute of Diabetes and Digestive and Kidney Disease, National Institutes of Health. 2010. Hemorrhoids. Publication No. 11–3021.

NIH Consensus Development Conference. 1994. *Helicobacter pylori* in peptic ulcer disease. *Journal of the American Medical Association* 272: 65–69.

Soll, A. H. 1996. Medical treatment of peptic ulcer disease. Practice guidelines. [Review]. European Helicobacter pylori. *Journal of the American Medical Association* 275: 622–29.

Study Group. 1997. Current European concepts in the management of H. pylori information. The Maastricht Consensus. *Gut* 41: 8–13.

Torpy, J., et al. 2010. Stomach Cancer. *Journal of the American Medical Association* 303(17): 1771.

U.S. Cancer Statistics Working Group. 2012. *United States Cancer Statistics: 1999–2008 Incidence and Mortality Web-based Report*. Atlanta, GA: Department of Health and Human Services, Centers for Disease Control and Prevention, and National Cancer Institute.

Wang, X., et al. 2009. Review of salt consumption and stomach cancer risk: Epidemiological and biological evidence. *World Journal of Gastroenterology* 15(18): 2204–13.

World Cancer Research Fund/American Institute for Cancer Research. 1997. Food research and the prevention of cancer: A global perspective. Washington, DC: American Institute for Cancer Research.

Yang, W.G., et al. 2011. A case-control study on the relationship between salt intake and salty taste and risk of gastric cancer. *World Journal of Gastroenterology* 17(15): 2049–53.

Chapter 9: Feeling Hormonal?

American Association of Clinical Endocrinologists Growth Hormone Task Force. 2003. American Association of Clinical Endocrinologists medical guidelines for clinical practice for growth hormone use in adults and children—2003 update. *Endocrine Practice* 9(1): 64–76.

American Cancer Society. 2011. Thyroid cancer. http://www.cancer.org/Cancer/ThyroidCancer/DetailedGuide/thyroid-cancer-survival-rates.

American Diabetes Association. 2011. *National Diabetes Fact Sheet*. January 2011.

American Diabetes Association. 2011. Standards of medical care in diabetes. 2011. *Diabetes Care* 34(Suppl. 1): S11–61.

Barres, R., et al. 2010. Acute exercise remodels promoter methylation in human skeletal muscle. *Cell Metabolism* 15(3): 405–11.

Blackwell, J., 2004. Evaluation and treatment of hyperthyroidism and hypothyroidism. *Journal of the American Academy of Nurse Practitioners* 16(10): 422–25.

Boyle, J. P., et al. 2010. Projection of the year 2050 burden of diabetes in the US adult population: Dynamic modeling of incidence, mortality, and prediabetes prevalence. *Population Health Metrics* 8: 29.

Centers for Disease Control and Prevention. 2010. *Number of Americans with Diabetes Projected to Double or Triple by 2050*. Press Release, October 22.

Centers for Disease Control and Prevention. 2011. *National Diabetes Fact Sheet*. January 2011, p. 11.

Cleveland Clinic. 2009. Thyroid Disease. http://my.clevelandclinic.org/disorders/hyperthyroidism/hic_thyroid_disease.aspx.

Cleveland Clinic. 2012. Thyroid cancer. http://my.clevelandclinic.org/disorders/thyroid_cancer/hic_thyroid_cancer.aspx.

Harvard School of Public Health. The nutrition source, simple steps to preventing diabetes. http://www.hsph.harvard.edu/nutritionsource/more/diabetes-fullstory/index.html#weight-control.

Hu, F. B., et al. 2001. Diet, lifestyle, and the risk of type 2 diabetes mellitus in women. *New England Journal of Medicine* 345: 790–97.

Laine, C., Wilson, J. F. 2007. Type 2 diabetes. *Annals of Internal Medicine* 146(1): ITC1–1.

Kapoor, D., and T. H. Jones. 2005. Smoking and hormones in health and endocrine disorders. *European Journal of Endocrinology* 152(4): 491–99.

Kelly, M. 2010. Supercharge your metabolism! *Fitness Magazine* (July/August).

Kochikuzhyil, B. M., et al. 2010. Effect of saturated fatty acid-rich dietary vegetable oils on lipid profile, antioxidant enzymes and glucose tolerance in diabetic rats. *Indian Journal of Pharmacology* 42(3): 142–45.

Levine, J. A., et al. 1999. Role of nonexercise activity thermogenesis in resistance to fat gain in humans. *Science* 283(5399): 212–14.

Mayo Clinic. 2011. Graves' disease. http://www.mayoclinic.com/health/graves -disease/DS00181/DSECTION=risk-factors.

Minaker, K. L. 2007. Common clinical sequelae of aging. In: Goldman, L., and Ausiello D, eds. *Cecil Medicine* 23rd edition

National Institute of Diabetes and Digestive and Kidney Diseases, National Institutes of Health. 2005. Diabetes, heart disease, and stroke. Publication No. 06-5094.

National Institute of Diabetes and Digestive and Kidney Diseases, National Institutes of Health. 2011. National Diabetes Statistics 2011. Publication No. 11-3892.

National Institutes of Health. 2010. Exercise and immunity. 2010. http://www.nlm .nih.gov/medlineplus/ency/article/007165.htm.

National Institutes of Health. 2011. Type 2 Diabetes Risk Factors. http://www.nlm .nih.gov/medlineplus/ency/article/002072.htm.

Norwegian University of Science and Technology. 2011. Feed your genes. http:// www.ntnu.edu/news/feed-your-genes.

Olshansky, S. J., and T. T. Perls. 2008. New developments in the illegal provision of growth hormone for "anti-aging" and bodybuilding. *Journal of the American Medical Association* 299(23): 2792–94.

Perls, T. T., et al. 2005. Provision or distribution of growth hormone for "antiaging" clinical and legal issues. *Journal of the American Medical Association* 294(16): 2086–90.

Sircar, S., and U. Kansra. 1998. Choice of cooking oils—myths and realities. *Journal of the Indian Medical Association* 96(10): 304–7.

Stan, M. N., and Bahn, R.S. 2010. Risk factors for development or deterioration of Graves' ophthalmopathy. *Thyroid, Official Journal of the American Thyroid Association* 20(7): 777–83.

Tweed, J. O., et al. 2012. The endocrine effects of nicotine and cigarette smoke. *Trends in Endocrinology and Metabolism* (May 2. Epub ahead of print).

University of Utah Health Care. 2003. Is eight enough? U researcher says drink up and tells why. News Archive.

U.S. Food and Drug Administration. 2007. Import alert 66-71, detention without physical examination of human growth hormone (HGH), also known as somatropin.

U.S. National Library of Medicine, National Institutes of Health. 2012. Aging changes in hormone production. http://www.nlm.nih.gov/medlineplus/ ency/article/004000.htm.

Weight Control Information Network, National Institutes of Health. 2004. Do you know the health risks of being overweight? Publication No. 07-4098.

Chapter 10: Make No Bones about It

American Academy of Orthopaedic Surgeons & American Orthopaedic Foot & Ankle Society. 2006. Tight shoes and foot problems. http://orthoinfo.aaos.org/topic.cfm?topic=A00146&return_link=0.

American Academy of Orthopedic Surgeons. May 2010. Smoking and Musculoskeletal Health. http://orthoinfo.aaos.org/topic.cfm?topic=A00192.

American Chiropractic Association. Today's fashion can be tomorrow's pain. http://www.acatoday.org/content_css.cfm?CID=73.

Bartlett, S. Osteoarthritis weight management. The Johns Hopkins Arthritis Center. http://www.hopkins-arthritis.org/patient-corner/disease-management/osteoandweight.html.

Centers for Disease Control and Prevention (CDC). 2006. Fatalities and injuries from falls among older adults—United States, 1993–2003 and 2001–2005. *MMWR Morbidity Mortality Weekly Report.* November 17; 55(45): 1221–24.

Cranney, A., et al. 2006. Clinical Guidelines Committee of Osteoporosis Canada. Parathyroid hormone for the treatment of osteoporosis: A systematic review. *Canadian Medical Association Journal* 175(1): 52–59.

Franks, A. L., et al. 1999. Encouraging news from the SERM frontier. *Journal of the American Medical Association* 281(23): 2243–44.

Gass, M., and B. Dawson-Hughes. 2006. Preventing osteoporosis-related fractures: An overview. *American Journal of Medicine* 119: S3–S11.

Hausdorff, J. M., et al., 2001. Gait variability and fall risk in community-living older adults: A 1-year prospective study. *Archives of Physical Medicine and Rehabilitation* 82(8): 1050–56.

Hollenbach, K. A., et al. 1993. Cigarette smoking and bone mineral density in older men and women. *American Journal of Public Health* 83(9): 1265–70.

Institute of Medicine of the National Academies. 2002/2005. Dietary reference intakes for energy, carbohydrate, fiber, fat, fatty acids, cholesterol, protein, and amino acids. http://www.iom.edu/Global/News%20Announcements/~/media/C5CD2DD7840 544979A549EC47E56A02B.ashx.

Management of osteoporosis in postmenopausal women: 2010 position statement of The North American Menopause Society. *Menopause* 17(1): 25–54.

National Institute of Arthritis and Musculoskeletal and Skin Diseases. 2010. Handout on Health: Osteoarthritis. *National Institutes of Health.* Publication No. 10-4617.

NIH Consensus Development Panel on Osteoporosis Prevention, Diagnosis, and Therapy. 2001. Osteoporosis prevention, diagnosis, and therapy. *Journal of the American Medical Association* 285(6): 785–95.

Rapuri, P. B., et al. 2000. Smoking and bone metabolism in elderly women. *Bone* 27(3): 429–36.

U.S. Department of Health & Human Services, Office of the Surgeon General. 2004. Bone health and osteoporosis: A report of the Surgeon General. *Reports of the Surgeon General.*

U.S. Department of Agriculture. 2012. Agriculture Research Service, National Agriculture Library. National Nutrient Database for Standard Reference.

U.S. National Library of Medicine and National Institutes of Health. 2011. Arm injuries and disorders. http://www.nlm.nih.gov/medlineplus/arminjuriesand disorders.html.

Waters, D. L., et al. 2000. Sarcopenia: Current perspectives. *Journal of Nutrition, Health, and Aging.* 4(3): 133–39.

Chapter 12: Still Sexy After All Those Years

American Cancer Society. 2011. Breast cancer.http://www.cancer.org/Cancer/Breast Cancer/DetailedGuide/breast-cancer-risk-factors.

American Cancer Society. 2011. Endometrial (uterine) cancer. http://www.cancer .org/Cancer/EndometrialCancer/DetailedGuide/endometrial-uterine -cancer-key-statistics.

American Cancer Society. 2011. Ovarian cancer. http://www.cancer.org/Cancer/ OvarianCancer/DetailedGuide/ovarian-cancerkey-statistics.

American Cancer Society. 2011. Women and smoking. http://www.cancer.org/ Cancer/CancerCauses/TobaccoCancer/WomenandSmoking/women-and -smoking-health-of-others.

American Council on Exercise. Exercise and menopause. http://www.acefitness.org/ fitfacts/fitfacts_display.aspx?itemid=91.

American Institute for Cancer Research. Foods that fight cancer. http://www.aicr .org/foods-that-fight-cancer/.

Bachmann, G. A., et al. 2000. Diagnosis and treatment of atrophic vaginitis. *American Family Physician* 61(10): 3090–96.

Beral, V., et al. 2008. Collaborative Group on Epidemiological Studies of Ovarian Cancer. Ovarian cancer and oral contraceptives: Collaborative reanalysis of data from 45 epidemiological studies including 23,257 women with ovarian cancer and 87,303 controls. *Lancet* 371(9609): 303–14.

Beral, V., et al. 2005. Endometrial cancer and hormone-replacement therapy in the Million Women Study. *Lancet* 365(9470): 1543–51.

Bianchini, F., et al. 2002. Overweight, obesity, and cancer risk. *Lancet Oncology*, 3(9): 565–74.

Chen, W. Y., et al. 2011. Moderate alcohol consumption during adult life, drinking patterns, and breast cancer risk. *Journal of the American Medical Association* 306(17): 1884–90.

Decahanet, C., et al. 2011. Effects of cigarette smoking on reproduction. *Human Reproduction Update* 17(1): 76–95.

Division of Cancer Prevention and Control, National Center for Chronic Disease Prevention and Health Promotion. 2010. Ovarian cancer risk factors. http://www.cdc.gov/cancer/ovarian/basic_info/risk_factors.htm.

Harvard Women's Health Watch. 2007. Pelvic organ prolapse can run in family. 14(9): 3.

Hull, M. G., et al. 2000. Delayed conception and active and passive smoking. The Avon Longitudinal Study of Pregnancy and Childhood Study Team. *Fertility and Sterility* 74(4): 725–33.

Jeng, C., et al. 2004. Menopausal women: Perceiving continuous power through the experience of regular exercise. *Journal of Clinical Nursing* 13(4): 447–54.

Krishnan, A. V., et al. 2012. The role of vitamin D in cancer prevention and treatment. *Rheumatic Diseases Clinics of North America* 38(1): 161–78.

Liu, R. H. 2004. Potential synergy of phytochemicals in cancer prevention: Mechanism of action. *Journal of Nutrition* 134(12 Suppl.): 3479S–85S.

Maeda, N., et al. 2011. Anti-cancer effect of spinach glycoglycerolipids as angiogenesis inhibitors based on the selective inhibition of DNA polymerase activity. *Mini Reviews in Medicinal Chemistry* 11(1): 32–38.

Mayo Clinic. 2011. Menopause. http://www.mayoclinic.com/health/menopause/ds00119/dsection=alternative-medicine.

Mayo Clinic. 2012. Premenstrual syndrome (PMS). http://www.mayoclinic.com/health/premenstrual-syndrome/ds00134/dsection=alternative-medicine.

National Cancer Institute. 2010. What you need to know about ovarian cancer. http://www.cancer.gov/cancertopics/wyntk/ovary/allpages.

Norman, R. J., et. al. 2004. Improving reproductive performance in overweight/obese women with effective weight management. *Human Reproductive Update* 10(3): 267–80.

Rocha Filho, E. A., et al. 2011. Essential fatty acids for premenstrual syndrome and their effect on prolactin and total cholesterol levels: A randomized, double blind, placebo-controlled study. *Reproductive Health* 8: 2.

Seitz, H. K., and P. Becker, 2007. Alcohol metabolism and cancer risk. *Alcohol Research & Health: Journal of the National Institute on Alcohol Abuse and Alcoholism* 30(1): 38–41.

Soares, S. R., and M. A. Melo. 2008. Cigarette smoking and reproductive function. *Current Opinion in Obstetrics & Gynecology* (June).

Sun, L., et al. 2012. Meta-analysis suggests that smoking is associated with an increased risk of early natural menopause. *Menopause* 19(2): 126–32.

U.S. Department of Agriculture. 2012. Agriculture Research Service, National Agriculture Library. National Nutrient Database for Standard Reference.

Villaverde-Gutierrez, C., et al. 2006. Quality of life of rural menopausal women in response to a customized exercise programme. *Journal of Advanced Nursing* 54(1): 11–19.

Walker, G.R., et al. 2002. Family history of cancer, oral contraceptive use, and ovarian cancer risk. *American Journal of Obstetrics and Gynecology* 186(1): 8–14.

Yao, L.H., 2004. Flavonoids in food and their health benefits. *Plant Foods for Human Nutrition* (Netherlands) 59(3): 113–22.

Zavos, P. 2000. Cigarette smoking and sexual health. American Council on Science and Health.

Ziaei, S., et al. 2007. The effect of vitamin E on hot flashes in menopausal women. *Gynecologic and Obstetric Investigation* 64(4): 204–7.

Chapter 13: Macho, Macho Man

Adam, O., et al. 2003. Anti-inflammatory effects of a low arachidonic acid diet and fish oil in patients with rheumatoid arthritis. *Rheumatology International* (1): 27–36.

American Cancer Society. 2012. Testicular cancer. http://www.cancer.org/Cancer/TesticularCancer/DetailedGuide/testicular-cancer-key-statistics.

Barry, M. J., et al. 2011. Effect of increasing doses of saw palmetto extract on lower urinary tract symptoms: A randomized trial. *Journal of the American Medical Association* 306(12): 1344–51.

Billups, K. L., et al. 2003. Relation of C-reactive protein and other cardiovascular risk factors to penile vascular disease in men with erectile dysfunction. *International Journal of Impotence Research* 15(4): 231–36.

Chavarro, J. E., et al. 2008. Soy food and isoflavone intake in relation to semen quality parameters among men from an infertility clinic. *Human Reproduction* 23(11): 2584–90.

Esposito, K., et al. 2005. High proportions of erectile dysfunction in men with the metabolic syndrome. *Diabetes Care* 28(5): 1201–3.

Hammadeh, M. E., et al. 2010. Protamine contents and P1/P2 ratio in human spermatozoa from smokers and non-smokers. *Human Reproduction* 25(11): 2708–20.

Institute of Medicine of the National Academies. 2002/2005. Dietary reference intakes for energy, carbohydrate, fiber, fat, fatty acids, cholesterol, protein, and amino acids. http://www.iom.edu/Global/News%20Announcements/~/media/C5CD2DD784544979A549EC47E56A02B.ashx.

Ma, R. C. W., and P. C. Y. Tong. 2010. Testosterone levels and cardiovascular disease. *Heart* 96: 1787–88.

Mamsen, L. S., et al. 2010. Cigarette smoking during early pregnancy reduces the number of embryonic germ and somatic cells. *Human Reproduction* 25(11): 2755–61.

Mason, E. 2010. Smoking damages men's sperm and also the numbers of germ and somatic cells in developing embryos. *European Society of Human Reproduction and Embryology*.

Mayo Clinic. 2012. Erectile dysfunction. http://www.mayoclinic.com/health/erectile-dysfunction/ds00162/dsection=risk-factors.

Mills, T. M. 2002. Vasoconstriction and vasodilatation in erectile physiology. *Current Urology Reports* 3(6): 477–83.

National Institute of Diabetes and Digestive and Kidney Diseases, National Institutes of Health. 2006. Prostate enlargement: Benign prostate hyperplasia. Publication No. 07–3012

National Institutes of Health (NIH) Consensus Conference. 1993. NIH Consensus Development Panel on Impotence. Impotence. *Journal of the American Medical Association* 270: 83–90.

Pittman, G. 2012. Sperm may feel the weight of extra pounds: Study. *Reuters Health*. http://www.reuters.com/article/2012/03/15/us-weight-idUSBRE82 E14820120315.

Sermondade, N., et al. 2012. Obesity and increased risk of oligozoospermia and azoospermia. *Archives of Internal Medicine* 172(5): 440–42.

Siepmann, T., 2011. Hypogonadism and erectile dysfunction associated with soy-product consumption. *Nutrition* 27(7–8): 859–62.

Simonsen, U., et al. 2002. Penile arteries and erection. *Journal of Vascular Research* 39(4): 283–303.

Suzuki, S., et al. 2002. Intakes of energy and macronutrients and the risk of benign prostatic hyperplasia. *American Journal of Clinical Nutrition* 75(4): 689–97.

Tivesten, A., et al. 2009. Low serum testosterone and estradiol predict mortality in elderly men. *Journal of Clinical Endocrinology and Metabolism* 94(7): 2482–88.

Travison, T. October 2006. Online Edition. News release, The Endocrine Society. *Journal of Clinical Endocrinology and Metabolism*.

U.S. National Library of Medicine, National Institutes of Health. 2011. Enlarged prostate. www.nlm.nih.gov/medlineplus/ency/article/000381.htm

U.S. National Library of Medicine, National Institutes of Health. 2011. Saw palmetto. http://www.nlm.nih.gov/medlineplus/druginfo/natural/971.html.

Chapter 14: Keep Your Stream Steady

8 Areas of Age-Related Change. 2007. *NIH Medline Plus* 2(1): 10–13. http://www.nlm .nih.gov/medlineplus/magazine/issues/winter07/articles/winter07pg10-13 .html.

American Cancer Society. 2012. Prostate cancer. http://www.cancer.org/Cancer/ ProstateCancer/DetailedGuide/prostate-cancer-key-statistics.

Ballard, A., and H. Richter. 2011. Impact of obesity and weight loss on urinary and bowel incontinence. *Menopausal Medicine* 9(3).

Brown, J. S., R. Wing, E. Barrett-Connor, et al. 2006. Diabetes Prevention Program Research Group. Life-style intervention is associated with lower prevalence of urinary incontinence: The Diabetes Prevention Program. *Diabetes Care* 29(2): 385–90.

Culligan, P., and M. Heit. 2000. Urinary incontinence in women: Evaluation and management. *American Family Physician* 62(11): 2433–44.

Curhan, G. C. 2011. Nephrolithiasis. In: Goldman L, Schafer AI, eds., *Cecil Medicine* 24th ed., chap 128.

Finkielstein, V. A. 2006. Strategies for preventing calcium oxalate stones. *Canadian Medical Association Journal* 174(10): 1407–9.

Gerber G. S., and C. B. Brendler. 2007. Evaluation of the urologic patient: History, physical examination, and the urinalysis. *Campbell-Walsh Urology*, 9th ed., chap. 3.

Grandwohl, S., et al. 2005. Urinary tract infection. *University of Michigan Health System*. http://cme.med.umich.edu/pdf/guideline/uti05.pdf.

Hansen, A., et al. 2011. Older persons and heat-susceptibility: The role of health promotion in a changing climate. *Health Promotion Journal of Australia* 22(Spec. No.): S17–20.

Jaipadkee, S., et al. 2004. The effects of potassium and magnesium supplements on urinary risk factors of renal stone patients. *Journal of the Medical Association of Thailand* 87(3): 255–63.

Kontiokari, T., et al. 2003. Dietary factors protecting women from urinary tract infection. *American Journal of Clinical Nutrition* 29(2): 266–69.

Makary, M. A., et al. 2012. The impact of obesity on urinary tract infection risk. *Urology* 79(2): 266–69.

Marieb, E. N. 1998. *Human Anatomy & Physiology*. Menlo Park, Calif.: Benjamin/Cummings.

Mayo Clinic. September 30, 2011. http://www.mayoclinic.com/health/urine-color/DS01026.

The Merck Manuals: The Merck Manual for Healthcare Professionals. 2008. Dehydration. http://www.merckmanuals.com/home/hormonal_and_metabolic_disorders/water_balance/dehydration.html.

National Institute of Diabetes and Digestive and Kidney Diseases, National Institutes of Health. 2006. Prostate enlargement: Benign prostatic hyperplasia. Publication No. 07-3012.

National Institute of Diabetes and Digestive and Kidney Diseases, National Institutes of Health. 2007. Urinary incontinence in women. Publication No. 08-4132.

National Institutes of Health of the U.S. Department of Health and Human Services. 2007. Your urinary system and how it works. Publication No. 07-3195.

National Kidney Foundation. 2012. Urinary tract infections. http://www.kidney.org/atoz/content/uti.cfm.

Nikolavsky, D., and M. Chancellor. 2009. Stress incontinence and prolapse therapy assessment. *Reviews in Urology* 11(1): 41–43.

Pietrow, P. K., and G. M. Preminger. 2007. Evaluation and medical management of urinary lithiasis. In: Wein, A. J., ed., *Campbell-Walsh Urology*, 9th ed. Philadelphia: Saunders Elsevier, chap 43.

Plowman, S. A., Smith, D.L. 2011. *Exercise Physiology for Health, Fitness and Performance*, 3rd ed. Philadelphia: Wolters Kluwer Health/Lippincott Williams & Wilkins.

Sheehy, C. M., et al. 1999. Dehydration: Biological considerations, age-related changes, and risk factors in older adults. *Biological Research for Nursing* 1(1): 30–37.

Spector, D. A. 2007. Urinary stones. *Principles of Ambulatory Medicine*, 7th ed., 754–66.

Subak, L. L., C. Johnson, E. Whitcomb, et al. 2002. Does weight loss improve incontinence in moderately obese women? *International Urogynecology Journal and Pelvic Floor Dysfunction* 13(1): 40–43.

Subak, L. L., E. Whitcomb, H. Shen, et al. 2005. Weight loss: A novel and effective treatment for urinary incontinence. *Journal of Urology* 174(1): 190–95.

U.S. National Library of Medicine, National Institutes of Health. 2011. Urinary Tract Infections—Adults. http://www.nlm.nih.gov/medlineplus/ency/article/000521.htm.

UT Southwestern Medical Center. 2004. Excess body weight linked to formation of uric acid kidney stones, UT Southwestern researchers find. http://www.utsouthwestern.edu/newsroom/news-releases/year-2004/excess-body-weight-linked-to-formation-of-uric-acid-kidney-stones-ut-southwestern-researchers-find.html.

Vulker, R. 1998. International group seeks to dispel incontinence "taboo." *Journal of the American Medical Association* 11: 951–53.

Yale Medical Group. Urinary tract infections (UTIs). http://www.yalemedicalgroup.org/stw/Page.asp?PageID=STW024091.

Zeegers, M. P., F. E. Tan, E. Dorant, and P. A. van Den Brandt. 2000. The impact of characteristics of cigarette smoking on urinary tract cancer risk: A meta-analysis of epidemiologic studies. *Cancer* 89(3): 630–39. http://www.ncbi.nlm.nih.gov/pubmed/10931463.

Chapter 16: Clearing the Air on Toxins

Alcaraz-Zubeldia, M., et al. 2008. The effect of supplementation with omega-3 polyunsaturated fatty acids on markers of oxidative stress in elderly exposed to PM. *Environmental Health Perspectives* 116(9).

Baldi, I., et al. 2011. Neurobehavioral effects of long-term exposure to pesticides: Results from the 4-year follow-up of the PHYTONER study. *Occupational and Environmental Medicine* 68(2): 108–15.

Bouchard, M. F., et. al. 2010. Attention-deficit/hyperactivity disorder and urinary metabolites of organophosphate pesticides. *Pediatrics* 6: e1270–77.

Bronstein, A. C., et al. 2009. 2008 Annual Report of the American Association of Poison Control Centers' National Poison Data System (NPDS): 26th Annual Report. *Clinical Toxicology* 47: 911–1084.

Centers for Disease Control and Prevention (US); National Center for Chronic Disease Prevention and Health Promotion (US); Office on Smoking and Health (US). 2010. How tobacco smoke causes disease: The biology of behavioral basis for smoking-attributable disease: *A Report of the Surgeon General.*

Environmental Working Group. Executive Summary, Shopper's Guide to Pesticides in Produce. http://www.ewg.org/foodnews/summary/.

Fang, Y. Z., et al. 2004. Glutathione metabolism and its implications for health. *Journal of Nutrition* 134(3): 489–92.

Feldman, J., et al. 2010. Wide range of diseases linked to pesticides. *Beyond Pesticides: Pesticides and You* 30(2).

Grodstein, F., et al. 2012. Exposure to particulate air pollution and cognitive decline inolder women. *Archives of Internal Medicine* 172(3): 219–27.

Hoek, G., et al., 2002. Association between mortality and indicators of traffic-related air pollution in the Netherlands: A cohort study. *Lancet* 360(9341): 1203–9.

Jafri, A. B. 2011. Aging and toxins. *Clinics in Geriatric Medicine* 24: 609–28.

Johns Hopkins Health Alert. 2006. Colonics: How risky are they? http://www.johns hopkinshealthalerts.com/alerts/digestive_health/JohnHopkinsHealth AlertsDigestiveDisorders_520-1.html.

Menzel, D. B. 1992. Antioxidant vitamins and prevention of lung disease. *Annals of the New York Academy of Sciences* 669: 141–55.

Moulton, P. V., and W. Yang. 2012. Air pollution, oxidative stress, and Alzheimer's disease. *Journal of Environmental and Public Health* 2012.

United States Environmental Protection Agency. The inside story: A guide to indoor air quality. http://www.epa.gov/iaq/pub/insidestory.html.

U.S. Environmental Protection Agency. 2009. Step It Up to Indoor AirPlus. EPA 402/ K-09/003.

Chapter 17: HOW You Live → How LONG You Live

Adit, A. 2009. Demographic differences and trends of vitamin D insufficiency in the US population, 1988–2004. *Archives of Internal Medicine* 169: 626–32.

Andres, G., et al. 2005. Effect of social networks on 10 year survival in very old Australians: The Australian longitudinal study of aging. *Journal of Epidemiology and Community Health* 59(7): 574–79.

Bennett, P., et al. March 30, 2011. Higher energy expenditure in humans predicts natural mortality. *Journal of Clinical Endocrinology & Metabolism*, jc. 2010–2944.

Brennan, F. X., and C. J. Charnetski. 2004. Sexual frequency and salivary immunoglobulin A (IgA).*Psychological Reports* 94(3) (Pt 1): 839–44.

Centers for Disease Control and Prevention (CDC). 2004. National Center for Health Statistics. Almost half of Americans use at least one prescription drug, annual report on nation's health shows. Press Release, December 2.

Crowe, M., et al. 2009. Personality and lifestyle in relation to dementia incidence. *Neurology* 72(3): 253–59.

Date, C., et al. 2009. Association of sleep duration with mortality from cardiovascular disease and other causes for Japanese men and women: The JACC study. *SLEEP* 32(3): 259–301.

Dietz, N., et al. 2007. Corporation for National and Community Service, Office of Research and Policy Development. The health benefits of volunteering: A review of recent research, Washington, DC.

Ebrahim, S., et al. 2002. Sexual intercourse and risk of ischaemic stroke and coronary heart disease: The Caerphilly study. *Journal of Epidemiology and Community Health* 56(2): 99–102.

Ehsani A. A., et al. 2006. Long-term caloric restriction ameliorates the decline in diastolic function in humans. *Journal of the American College of Cardiology* 47(2): 398–402.

Emmons, R. A., and M. E. McCuiloug. 2003. Counting blessings versus burdens: An experimental investigation of gratitude and subjective well-being in daily life. *Journal of Personality and Social Psychology* 84(2): 377–89.

Frankel, S., et al. 1997. Sex and death: Are they related? Findings from the Caerphilly cohort study. *British Medical Journal* 315: 1641.

Garfinkel, L., et al. 2002. Mortality associated with sleep duration and insomnia. *Achieves of General Psychiatry* 59(2).

George, L. K., et al. 2000. Spirituality and health: What we know, what we need to know. *Journal of Social and Clinical Psychology* 19(1); Psychology Module.

Giovannucci, E., et al. 2004. Ejaculation frequency and subsequent risk of prostate cancer. *Journal of the American Medical Association* 291(13): 1578–86.

Glaser, R., et al., 1988. Disclosure of traumas and immune function: Health implications for psychotherapy. *Journal of Consulting and Clinical Psychology* 56(2): 239–45.

Holt-Lunstad, J., et al. 2010. Social relationships and mortality risk: A meta-analytic review. *PLoS Med* 7(7): e1000316. doi:10.1371/journal.pmed.1000316.

Kim, E. S., et al. 2011. Dispositional Optimism Protects Older Adults from Stroke. *Stroke Magazine* (July).

Kirshnit, C., and D. McClelland. 1998. The effect of motivational arousal through films on salivary immunoglobulin A. *Psychology and Health* 2: 31–52.

Lutgendorf, S. K., et al. 2005. Social support, psychological distress, and natural killer cell activity in ovarian cancer. *American Society of Clinical Oncology* 23(28): 7105–13.

Memon, M. Z., et al. 2009. Car ownership and the risk of fatal cardiovascular diseases. Results from the second national health and nutrition examination study mortality follow-up study. *Journal of Vascular and Interventional Neurology* 2(1): 132–35.

Appendix

American Cancer Society. 2012. Guide to quitting smoking. Healthy living information to help you stay well. http://www.cancer.org/Healthy/StayAwayfrom Tobacco/GuidetoQuittingSmoking/.

American Council on Exercise. 2012. Exercise Library. ACE get fit. http://www.ace fitness.org/exerciselibrary/default.asp&xgt.

American Heart Association. 2011. Quit smoking. Getting healthy. http://www .heart.org/HEARTORG/GettingHealthy/QuitSmoking/Quit-Smoking_UCM _001085_SubHomePage.jsp.

American Lung Association. How to quit smoking. http://www.lung.org/stop -smoking/how-to-quit/.

Baldauf, S. Salt intake: 14 heart numbers you should know about. *U.S. News*, n.d., Health. http://health.usnews.com/health-news/family-health/slideshows/ your-heart-health-14–numbers-everyone-should-know/4.

Barbella, L., and L. Mihelich. Unexpected sources lead to high sodium diet. *Times of Northwest Indiana* [Munster], March 3, 2012, n.p. http://www .nwitimes.com/lifestyles/home-and-garden/unexpected-sources-lead-to -high-sodium-diet/article_b08e917e-aae5-5e90-8e40-fdc59d3305d5.html.

Birklbauer, Walter. 2011. *Why Laughter Yoga? or The Guitar Method: A neurologic view.*

Centers for Disease Control. Vegetable of the month: Carrot. http://www.fruitsand veggiesmatter.gov/month/carrot.html.

Centers for Disease Control and Prevention. Quit smoking. Smoking and tobacco use. http://www.cdc.gov/tobacco/quit_smoking/.

Centers for Disease Control and Prevention. Target maximum heart rate and estimate maximum heart rate. Physical activity for everyone. n.d. http:// www.cdc.gov/physicalactivity/everyone/measuring/heartrate.html.

Cleveland Clinic. Quitting smoking. Treatments and procedures. http://my .clevelandclinic.org/services/Smoking_Cessation.

Gelfand, J. Abdominal exercises. Fitness and exercise. WebMD, LLC, March 27, 2010. http://www.webmd.com/fitness-exercise/guide/health-fitness-abs.

Juhan, B. Building healthy families. North Carolina State University. August 16, 2004, n.p. Accessed 2012. http://www.ces.ncsu.edu/montgomery/news letters/FCS/FCSaug04.html.

Kataria, M. 2002. *Laugh For No Reason* (2d ed.). Mumbai, India: Madhuri International.

Mayo Clinic. Balance exercises. Fitness. December 1, 2009. http://www.mayoclinic .com/health/balance-exercises/SM00049&slide=3.

Mayo Clinic. Sodium: How to tame your salt habit now. Nutrition and healthy eating. March 30, 2011. http://www.mayoclinic.com/health/sodium/NU00284.

National Cancer Institute. Quit guide. Smokefree.gov. http://www.smokefree.gov/.

PureHealthMD. Balance Exercises. Diet and fitness. Discovery fit and health, n.d. http://health.howstuffworks.com/wellness/diet-fitness/exercise/balance -exercises.htm.

Smoking Cessation Health Center. Quit smoking. WebMD, LLC. http://www
    .webmd.com/smoking-cessation/default.htm.

University of Georgia. Unexpected sources of sodium: Where is it coming from?
    Foods and Nutrition Education. June 2011. http://www.fcs.uga.edu/ext/
    pubs/fdns/FDNS-E-89-59a.pdf.

USDA. USDA National Nutrient Database for Standard Reference. National Agricul-
    tural Library. December 1, 2011. http://ndb.nal.usda.gov/.

INDEX

About the Author

Dr. Michael Rafael Moreno, better known as Dr. Mike, is a graduate of the University of California at Irvine and Hahnemann Medical School (now Drexel University). Following his residency at Kaiser Permanente in Fontana, California, Dr. Mike moved to San Diego, where he now practices family medicine and sits on the board of the San Diego Chapter of the American Academy of Family Physicians. In 2008, Dr. Mike launched "Walk with Your Doc," which he participates in every Tuesday and Thursday morning before his workday begins. The program began when Dr. Mike offered to walk with a patient to motivate her to exercise and has since grown into a thriving community. Dr. Mike takes pride in being viewed not only as a doctor but also as a friend and confidant.